GOING
the DISTANCE

THE THREE ESSENTIAL ELEMENTS OF
OPTIMAL LIFELONG FITNESS AND INJURY PREVENTION

By Cris Dobrosielski CSCS, CPT

Chris,
It is a privilege to watch you
grow. Keep going!

Train smart, have fun
and Never ever Give-up!

Coach Cris

Cris Dobrosielski

ISBN: 1481178172
ISBN-13: 9781481178174

Cris Dobrosielski is a nationally recognized expert in the fields of fitness, strength and conditioning, and injury prevention. Over the last three decades, he has helped thousands of individuals improve their health and their lives as a coach, guide and personal trainer. Athletes at the high school, collegiate and professional levels have benefited from his understanding of performance improvement and injury prevention. In his roles as associate head strength and conditioning coach at University of California San Diego (UCSD) and as head track and field and cross country coach at Cuyamaca Community College in Rancho San Diego, Cris maximized athletic potential and developed champions. In addition to his work with competitive athletes, he also served as an instructor for the Faculty/Staff Wellness Program at UCSD, as a physical education instructor at Cuyamaca Community College and as a personal trainer to cancer, stroke and cardiac patients. In 2012, he was hired by the American Council on Exercise (ACE) to serve as featured trainer and host for multiple educational videos that help to inspire and educate personal trainers around the world.

Cris holds certifications from ACE and the National Strength and Conditioning Association (NSCA). He is an honors graduate of San Diego State University, where, as a member of the Division I Varsity Cross-Country Team, he received the Western Athletic Conference Scholar/Athlete Award in his final semester. He has been a featured expert on CBS National News and is a frequent contributor to multiple San Diego television news stations including NBC7, as well as the *San Diego Union-Tribune*. He also writes regularly on injury prevention, athletic longevity and fitness motivation for *California Surf News Magazine*.

As an accomplished Masters athlete, Cris continues to compete and win at the highest levels nationally and internationally. He has won four age group World Championships, two National Championships and thirteen Southern California Regional Championships in swimming, paddleboarding, and surf lifesaving.

Cris lives in San Diego, California and is the owner and lead clinician at Monumental Results Fitness and Wellness Center in the community of Mission Hills.

Acknowledgements

There is an old Buddhist proverb that says, "When the student is ready, the teacher will appear." My life confirms this truth. At every point in my personal journey when I have needed guidance and insight, guidance and insight have appeared. Since *Going the Distance* is a book about building strong foundations, I want to particularly thank those individuals who were most influential in helping me build my foundation as an athlete and a person early in life.

First, there were the lifeguards of Salisbury State Beach and the bouncers at the Frolics Rock and Roll Ballroom in Massachusetts, just months after the death of my dad when I was 9 years old. Although many people played very important roles in my life at that time, there were three in particular whose mentorship helped shape my future path, the Big Three: "Wolfie" Simmons, Patrick Griffin and Craig Weir. These generous giants saw a boy who desperately needed a dad, and each in his own way stepped in and taught me lessons in self-reliance, self-defense, loyalty and friendship. Their love made me feel safe, the most important thing a child needs.

A few years later, as a scholarship student at the Governor's Academy, the oldest boarding school in the nation, I found myself in a dark and lonely adolescent tailspin. In the midst of that turbulent time, in walked three teachers who gave their counsel and their friendship. The unique relationship I had with each of them changed the course of my life: Steve Shea, Paul Wann and Elizabeth Ruhl saw beyond my agitation, frustration and inconsistency. The discussions, the tenderness and, most importantly, the example they set as people revealed to me alternative and healthier ways to view the world and my role in it. I learned about the satisfaction that comes from service and the healing power of self-expression.

These six people, and many others in my adult life, have each shown up at precisely the right time. Each has helped me become a better teacher, a better coach and a better man. For that, I am forever grateful.

I dedicate this book to my mother, Helen Elizabeth Dobrosielski.
Her life is an example of love, dedication and persistence.

Thank you, Mom. I love you.

Table of Contents

Author's Foreword

I have written *Going the Distance* to educate, encourage and promote the essential strategies one needs for developing optimal lifelong fitness and performance. It is my aim to present the most important and foundational ideas and techniques for athletic longevity, peak performance and injury prevention. I believe the information and techniques outlined in this book are beneficial and relevant for all athletes, across all sports, at every ability level. The plan that I present in this book can serve as a blueprint for developing and fortifying an approach to exercising, training and racing that is safe, sustainable, and supported by contemporary scientific research. Executing the plan outlined in this book will help the fitness enthusiast bypass pitfalls that are common in many well-intentioned training routines. The techniques presented in this book are foundational, and they are as useful to the elite athlete as they are to the novice. If your goal is to play the sports and participate in the fitness activities you love for as long as you can with fewer orthopedic interruptions, the techniques and philosophies of *Going the Distance* are crucial for your journey. If you are willing to make small but significant changes in the way you maintain your body and organize your workouts, *Going the Distance* will have a tremendous impact on your life.

My friend, basketball legend Bill Walton, has shared many interesting stories with me about one of his heroes, his basketball coach at UCLA, the great John Wooden. According to Bill, "Coach's" teaching and much of his success centered on his unyielding commitment to strong fundamentals, and on his young students building solid foundations on which advanced skills could be developed. The legendary coach's first bit of instruction for his basketball players was in putting on their socks and tying their sneakers properly to avoid the blistering and foot irritations that could sideline them. His attention to detail and foundation set a tone that he replicated in every area of team development.

In a similar fashion, this book is the first step to building a detail-oriented routine that addresses the demands your sport or hobby places on your body. As part of that first step, I invite you to learn the three essential elements to sustained and optimal lifelong fitness:

- Flexibility
- Core and major joint stability
- Proper recovery

These elements are best introduced in the context of a proper warm-up and a proper cool-down. Along with strength training and strategic and balanced cross-training, these three elements are part of what I call the Five Pillars of Lifelong Fitness™. I have chosen to focus on the first three pillars in this book because I believe they have the greatest potential to significantly impact athletic longevity, and for that reason they are at the foundation of my Five Pillars philosophy. They also represent the most logical, sequential starting point for athletes to begin changing the way they approach their fitness and athletic training. Understanding and implementing the first three pillars will help athletes and fitness enthusiasts better regulate safe levels of training frequency, intensity and volume.

A small encyclopedia could be written about each of the Five Pillars. In this book, I will identify and explain only the most important aspects of each of the three foundational pillars and the most practical and efficient methods of addressing them in your fitness routine.

My hope is that *Going the Distance* provides a specific yet customizable road map that will help you sustain your participation in sports and fitness activities throughout your life. The techniques and instructions contained in this book are based on the most current scientific literature, my long-term clinical experience as a coach, and the lessons I have learned from decades of athletic competition and training. The balanced and gradually progressive approach in this book is in contrast to many "one-size-fits-all," "no-pain, no-gain" models that make the same aggressive recommendations to forty-five-year-olds as they do to twenty-year-olds. The exercises I have selected are the starting point for building strong foundations in flexibility, stability and recovery. As you develop mastery over these exercises and techniques, it will be important to progressively and creatively introduce your body to different versions and more advanced techniques.[1]

The good news is that any improvement in your commitment to these three pillars will yield results. The more consistent your commitment, the more significant and predictable your results. By developing your flexibility and stability and committing to a balanced recovery process, you will greatly increase the possibility of achieving vibrant lifelong fitness. Furthermore, consistent dedication to this approach will decrease the likelihood and frequency of injuries.

I encourage you to aim for perfect adherence to the principles prescribed in this book, with the caveat that although perfection is a noble goal, doing the best you can is a great start.

I have experienced success in many areas of my life disproportionate to my natural abilities. My effort, persistence and commitment to learning have been at the center of all of my most significant achievements. That effort and attitude have helped me form my personal motto:

---

1 Advanced options will be the topic of a forthcoming book in the Five Pillars Series™ and will be systematically made available on my website, GoingtheDistancebook.com. I encourage you to visit regularly for advanced pointers, videos and coaching tips on training smarter.

Small consistent change, over a significant period of time, leads to monumental results.

Let the journey begin.

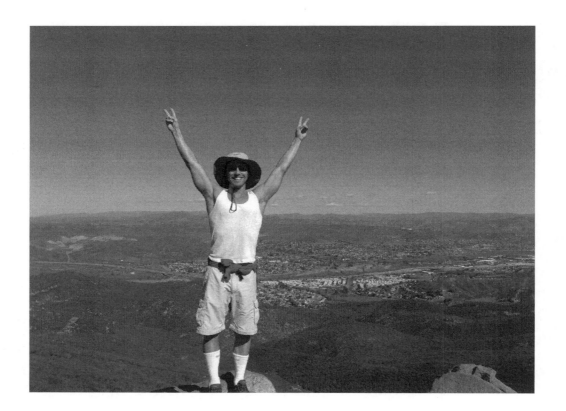

Introduction

A person can be as great as he wants to be. If you believe in yourself and have the courage, the determination, the dedication, the competitive drive and if you are willing to sacrifice the little things in life and pay the price for the things that are worthwhile, it can be done.

—Vince Lombardi

It is August, 2009. I'm at the United States Lifesaving Association National Championships in Fort Lauderdale, Florida. This is a three-day competition where the best ocean lifeguard athletes in the country gather to determine the fastest and fittest in their field. The events include short- and long-distance running, swimming, paddleboarding, surf skiing, and dory racing. All of the events tap into skills and techniques used in emergency rescue situations by ocean lifeguards. More than a thousand athletes typically compete in three to eight races a day, with most races ranging in duration from five to fifteen minutes. Each event begins with an open division race with no age restrictions that involves multiple qualifying heats, followed by age-specific races, each of which usually consists of one championship finals race. Until a competitor is thirty years old, he or she can only compete in gender-specific open division races. In my early and mid-thirties, I took the challenge energetically and competed in both age-specific and open races, with considerable success. In 2005, while competing in both types of races, I finished ninth in the open paddleboard race in Virginia Beach, Virginia. In 2006, I won a national championship in the 35-to-39 age group paddleboard race; in 2008, I qualified for two open division finals—meaning that I was one of the fifteen fastest racers in the nation—while also squeaking out a bronze medal in my age group's paddleboard race.

Now, as a forty-year-old athlete, I was once again confronting a nearly decade-old dilemma: how to balance my desire to compete in both age group and open events. This decision required me to weigh my drive to compete at my highest possible level against my hopes of staying injury-free. Should I participate in the age-specific events only, where my greatest chance of victory and lowest chance of injury lay, or should I also tackle some open events? The open events are the most prestigious and competitive races, with the winners declared the nation's best lifeguard athletes.

Adding open events to my schedule would exponentially increase my energy expenditure, and, as a result, my likelihood of debilitating fatigue or maybe even injury, which could severely impact my performance in the age-specific races. However, participating in both age-specific and open races is part of the challenge that makes this sport so much fun for me. In athletics, as in life, I've always derived great pleasure from stretching my personal limits. Ever since I completed my first 10k race, at the age of nine, the natural high of training, competing and pushing myself has been my healthy alternative to other forms of stress relief. Walking the razor's edge, weaving in and out of the lunatic fringe in my athletic endeavors, and accomplishing things people told me I couldn't achieve have always been medicine for my restless spirit. But like any medicine, too much at the wrong time can lead to unforeseen consequences.

In the months leading up to this competition, I had experienced some significant lower back pain after early season races, but my personal discipline and professional background had helped me manage this moderate irritation rather well. Although I had soreness and achiness, they never stopped me from competing: at the regional championships just two weeks earlier, I participated in ten events over eight hours and held up under the pressure. My athletic performance was not perfect, nor was it painless, but like many athletes and exercise enthusiasts, my perception of pain was obscured by my love of sport and desire to participate.

In the weeks before what would be a grueling experience in Fort Lauderdale, I had diligently considered what my appropriate level of participation should be. My goal was to maximize the thrill, challenge, and fun, while stopping short of injury. As I did my warm-up paddle on the racecourse at the National Championships on my first day of competition, I considered both my race strategy and the schedule I had set for the next two days. Normally I would not be second-guessing a plan this late, but I had to consider all the factors that could affect my ability to compete: a mild yet noticeable ache in my lower back, the excessive heat and humidity of summertime Florida, and the multiple days of racing ahead.

While I was finishing my higher-intensity pre-race warm-up on my paddleboard, the sun peeked through the heavy black clouds, which had just unloaded two inches of rain in less than thirty minutes. My adrenaline and enthusiasm increased with each stroke and my body became looser and more comfortable, signs of a good warm-up. The sun, still low in the eastern sky, was now out from behind the black clouds, and it seemed to encourage me to trust my training and follow through with my plan for a full schedule of both age group and open races. As I headed back to shore, I spotted my younger paddleboard competitors gathering for the start on the beach; most were ten to twenty years my junior. Excitement buzzed through my body, and my spirit rose. The opportunity to demonstrate my preparation and will seemed a magnificent blessing. I was once again thankful for this liberating annual ritual of stretching my limits, a ritual that had been part of my life for the past three decades.

All paddleboard courses at this national event, open and age group, are approximately a thousand meters, which is a little over a half-mile long. Each racer sprints into the water with a ten and-a-half-foot paddleboard under one arm, launches himself on the board and onto the water, knees down, and paddles furiously into the oncoming surf. The course is typically a triangle with an apex buoy. In the open paddleboard event, approximately one hundred racers fold into six heats. After the quarterfinal and semifinal heats, a final race of the sixteen remaining athletes is held late in the afternoon, as well as all of the other open division finals for the day's other events. The challenge for all athletes who compete in the open paddleboard is to make it to the finals while limiting energy expenditure in the preliminary qualifying rounds. This challenge was exacerbated for me, since I chose to compete not only in the two open qualifying rounds, but also in the age group finals held immediately after my second qualifying heat in the open.

With a Herculean effort, I squeaked out a bronze medal in the age group paddleboard finals race against the fastest forty-year-olds in the US. Inside of an hour, I raced again in the International Ironman. Enthusiasm was my primary fuel source, as the races had begun to significantly tap into my physical energy. I battled it out with Bruce Wilke, a fierce and experienced competitor from Hollywood Beach, FL, who probably had at least ten National Championships on his resume. The International Ironman lasted about twenty minutes and involved running, swimming, paddleboarding and surf ski racing. After going head-to-head in the run and the paddleboard sections, I made my move in the swim portion of the event and put just a couple seconds between me and the rest of the field. With my competitors in close pursuit, I reached down deep in the tank, hung on to my lead in the final surf ski leg and earned a National Championship. At this point, I was one hundred percent on track to achieve all my goals for that day—my plan was working. After medaling in the age group paddleboard, qualifying in the open paddleboard and winning the crown jewel, the Ironman, I was filled with satisfaction and pride.

While I waited for the paddleboard finals in the afternoon, I stretched, hydrated, and did a number of self-care techniques to relax my body and stay ready. The biggest difficulty was to remain cool in the high heat and humidity of a south Florida summer afternoon. Several hours passed until the moment finally arrived. As I stood beside my fellow competitors on the berm, just above the ocean's edge, I felt a sense of humility and excitement at the day's accomplishments. I also felt grateful to all the people over all the years who had been part of my involvement in this beautiful sport. For me, racing has always been as much about the process of preparing and the relationships with my teammates and competitors as it is about winning or losing.

I was, however, keenly aware of the massive energetic cost of all of my racing that morning, and also aware of the cumulative fatigue on my lower back. By afternoon, most competitors are somewhat beaten up from the morning races, but we are trained to manage this feeling—it is part of the thrill. It's at this point, with the final competition waiting, that one might argue that the challenge really begins.

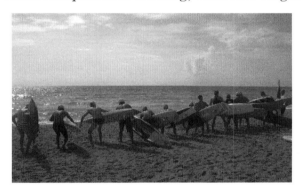 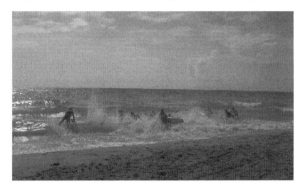

The starting gun sounded with a crack. As I charged into the water, my back tightened up almost immediately, and my left hamstring cramped. The heat of the day and the fatigue from the morning races had caught up with me much quicker than I had expected. I fought hard but knew right away that my body wasn't going to cooperate at the necessary level. I gave it my best, but despite my efforts, a back-of-the-pack finish was the best I could do. Though disappointed, I carried my board across the finish line with class and dignity, keeping in mind the motto my high school cross country coach David Abusarmra had taught me nearly twenty-five years earlier: "No matter what, always finish like a champion." All paddleboard races end with feelings of pain and exhaustion that quickly pass. What I felt in that moment was different, and I would later discover that it was not going away anytime soon.

I thought I had made a reasonable choice. I had surveyed the scene and worked out my plan, and I stand by my decision to have taken that monumental challenge. The thrill and the accomplishment of earning my spot in the finals and medaling were satisfying, but I would pay the price for many months with a constant radiating pain in my lumbar spine.

On the second day of racing, the bright tropical sunrise of Surfside, Florida served as my alarm clock. Unfortunately, the same pain and soreness were present in my back, but I still assumed they would subside. I was able to participate in the second day of competition, but my back was a limiting factor. I regulated my effort and intensity and was able to race four times and earn a bronze medal in the Run-Swim-Run.

When I returned to San Diego, I expected that ice, rest and time would heal my back, but I was wrong. Despite my attentiveness to my injury, it lingered for days, and then weeks. Very low-intensity exercise, self-care, and regular massage therapy were insufficient; the pain persisted and actually increased.

As summer turned to fall and fall to winter, the pain escalated until many daily activities, such as sitting, bending, and simple twisting, were uncomfortable. Despite my commitment to extensive physical therapy and a rehabilitation program, I made little progress. It seemed that the damage might be permanent. At some point in the recovery process, my ambition went from returning to high-intensity training and racing to simply living without pain. I worked tirelessly on my rehabilitation. After two subpar experiences at rehab clinics, I tracked down Stewart Sanders, an expert physical therapist and fellow athlete. He understood that it was more than just my back on the line, and he really poured out his care and skills. With Stewart's help, a targeted self-care routine, and months of rehabilitation, the constant pain incrementally diminished. I began to see the possibility of a pain-free back and the potential to return to competitive athletics at some level.

I knew, however, that recovery would be a long journey, and that from that moment forward, I would need to incorporate a mindfulness and maturity of decision-making that matched my enthusiasm for hard training. It was at this point that I began to see not only the importance, but the necessity, of utilizing my Five Pillars philosophy. I had come to a transition in my life. If I were to continue to stretch my physical limits through racing, my preparation and my attentiveness to my body's feedback would have to operate at a higher level. Not some of the time, but all of the time.

It is important to note that sometimes the perspective we use to regulate our choices is based on old, obsolete data. It is the responsibility of the athletes themselves, especially high-intensity competitive athletes, to acknowledge and account for the changes that occur in their bodies and their lives, changes that affect their ability to perform. That does not mean that we should roll over and accept every ache or pain as a limitation, but it does mean that we must address them so that we can fortify the raw materials that allow us to do what we do.

With that in mind, let's discuss the first crucial tool for addressing my first two Pillars, Flexibility and Stability: Proper Warm-Up. If followed closely, this formula will deliver results, provided you never stop thinking for yourself and always listen to your body.

Chapter One:
Warm-Up

Many aging athletes want to simply carry on the routine they were familiar with in their high school or college days. Even though they may be in good shape, they forget that their bodies are different and need more time and attention to safely prepare for strenuous exercise. Those who don't respect the natural changes that occur as we age are the same ones keeping me in business.

—Paul Stricker, MD, Sports Medicine and Olympic Physician

Many athletes and fitness enthusiasts do warm-up to some degree, but very few do so thoroughly or correctly. Consistently executing a gradually progressive warm-up is a key ingredient to maximizing the positive results of a workout and minimizing the likelihood of injury. A sport-specific warm-up is even more important when the workout includes high-intensity training. Along with a proper cool-down, many fitness professionals consider proper warm-up to be one of the two most important components of long-term success, especially for older athletes. Many of the strains, sprains and tears that often occur in high-intensity practices and games can be sidestepped or minimized if the athlete does a thorough warm-up and deliberately assesses the readiness of his or her body.

Metaphorically speaking, the human body is a lot like an automobile in terms of performance and maintenance requirements. If you have lived through a winter in a cold-weather climate, as I did growing up in Methuen, Massachusetts, then you know you can't expect good performance from your vehicle immediately after starting it, especially if it's an older model. If you were to put the car into drive and floor it, the ride would likely be rough and jerky, because the mixture of fuel and air would not be in equilibrium yet. The same is true of the human body. A warm-up's primary physiological purposes are to increase body temperature; lubricate joints; activate, stimulate and oxygenate muscles; and increase heart rate and breath rate. Beginning an activity without thoroughly warming up significantly reduces the workout's potential benefit and increases the possibility of injury. The primary reason is that the lack of warm-up results in lower physiological functioning—that is, heart rate, breathing, and oxygenation of muscles—which makes it more difficult, if not impossible, to train at your highest level. Every practice or training session is an opportunity to improve skill acquisition and fitness level. The latter requires high-intensity training that can be difficult for an athlete, especially an aging athlete, to achieve for a variety of reasons. Failure to warm up thoroughly can thus have a profound impact on your ability to train effectively. Over time, that means many training sessions do not reach their highest possible level, high-intensity activity, which is where important incremental fitness development occurs. Such missed opportunities can lead to a sustained performance plateau, which results in a lack of progress.

A warm-up is also a crucial ingredient in preparing an athlete's mental focus for a training session or competition. Time spent doing a gradually progressive warm-up helps create a transition from whatever you were doing prior to your workout to the precious time available that you have set aside for exercise. In particular, the general aerobic portion of a warm-up allows you to temporarily leave the worries of the day behind and experience the joy and release of physical activity. Time spent moving at relatively low intensity can help center the mind and ground the body in the present activity. This intentional act of connecting the mind and the body and being "in the moment," or ITM as I call it, decreases the likelihood of mental mistakes that often lead to injuries such as rolled ankles and twisted knees.

The third key benefit of a warm-up is its value as an assessment tool for evaluating your relative readiness for the workout at hand. A warm-up provides information about your energy level and shines a light on any physiological weak links, which might require more preparation before proceeding with more rigorous training. Such information allows you to adjust the volume and intensity of your workout to safely meet the needs of your body and to set realistic expectations for the training session. For instance, a hiker who planned to do an excessively hilly route could bypass a potential setback by switching to a more moderate route when she feels a twinge in her hamstring during the early warm-up phase. Similarly, the swimmer who planned to work on his butterfly stroke might extend the warm-up, do some additional dry land stretching, or reconsider the amount of "fly" to be done that day when he gets the message early on that his shoulders are irritated or tired.

Let's look more closely at the three aspects of a proper warm-up:
- General warm-up
- Dynamic stretching
- Sports-specific movements that progress gradually

Warm-up Element One: General Warm-Up

The first element of a general warm-up consists of low-intensity aerobic exercises. Some of my favorites are traditional movement patterns such as jogging, stationary cycling, low-intensity calisthenics and core stability exercises. With the exception of stationary cycling, none of the modes I mentioned above require any equipment. I also favor less-familiar movement patterns: skipping and variations of traditional calisthenics, such as Jumping Jacks, to add variety and neurological benefits to a traditional warm-up.

In choosing your general warm-up, consider safety, sport specificity, and a healthy balance of differing movement patterns. When contemplating safety issues, common sense is the rule. For instance, it is unwise for a barefooted swimmer to do a significant number of Jumping Jacks on a concrete pool deck. A better choice for him would be core body exercise on a towel, kickboard or stretching mat. Common sense also applies when thinking about sport specificity and a balance of movement patterns. The skipping series described below is excellent for basketball, because its movement patterns complement and mimic many of the movements of the game. On the other hand, for a kayaker or surfer, the same skipping series is beneficial because the upright, vertically loading positions of skipping, with feet planted in the earth, build strong bones and joints and are quite different from the movement and loading patterns in those sports. I encourage variety in your warm-up exercises to give your mind and body various forms of general aerobic stimulation and a positive physiological stress.

Let's review some of your options for the General Aerobic portion of your Warm-Up.

Skipping Series

Skipping is a low-intensity but dynamic plyometric exercise. Any form of skipping serves the purpose of a general warm-up, but being attentive to some basic mechanics will reinforce appropriate postures for most upright sports and for posture in general throughout your day.

You are best served by skipping in a relaxed, rhythmic fashion, with little elevation off of the ground. The skips I recommend are not hops and don't include jumping, but instead involve more of a gentle bounce or a shuffling movement pattern with minimal effort.

Proper Posture for Skipping

- Weight on balls of the feet
- Knees slightly bent
- Hips aligned on top of your heels or slightly forward
- Torso long and extended
- Shoulders relaxed
- Chest broad
- Chin neutral, not tilted up or down
- Jaw relaxed
- Crown of the head (upper back part of the skull) held high

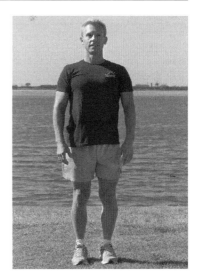

There are several different movement patterns of the upper body that you can do in conjunction with skipping. The four patterns below are some of my favorites and add neurological complexity and an upper-body flexibility benefit to the move.

- Opposite arm, opposite leg

- Both arms across the chest

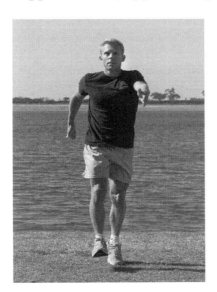

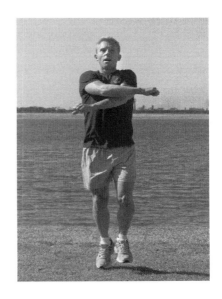

• Both arms backward

• Both arms overhead

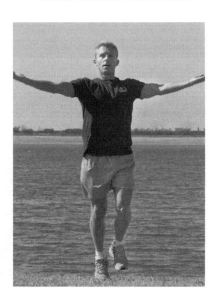

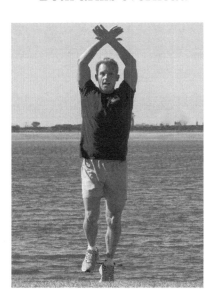

PROGRAM DESIGN FOR SKIPPING SERIES

- Two 20-yard repetitions of each of the four arm patterns

- Rest 5 to 10 seconds between each repetition

- Intensity is low but builds gradually

Jumping Jack Series

Assuming you have no acute injuries that would be irritated by the impact, Jumping Jacks are an excellent option for a general warm-up. Like skipping, they require no equipment and very little space. Also like skipping, this vertical loading technique can be an excellent sport-specific activity for any athlete, particularly one who plays court sports. In contrast to their sport-specific benefit, with proper footwear or a cushioned surface, Jumping Jacks can be an effective body balancing tool for aquatic athletes and those who get little vertical load on their feet, legs, hips and spine from their sport.

Jumping Jacks should be done with low intensity and should be few in number, with a focus on good form. Intensity, tempo and size of the Jumping Jack can increase as the warm-up continues and as you progress.

Proper Posture and Starting Position for Jumping Jacks

- Arms by your side, feet together
- Weight mostly on balls of feet
- Knees slightly bent
- Hips in vertical alignment with heels
- Torso extended
- Chest broad
- Shoulders back but relaxed
- Chin neutral
- Crown of the head high

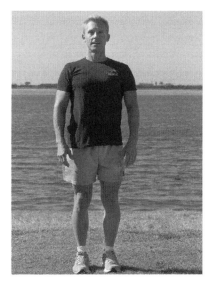

Begin by jumping your feet apart 6 to 12 inches as you swing your arms out and up to shoulder height. As your body warms up, gradually jump your feet wider and swing your arms to a nearly overhead position. Continue to maintain proper posture and eventually move into full jumping, where, assuming no shoulder pain, your arms are fully above your head and your legs are 12 to 24 inches apart.

You can increase the intensity of this exercise form by trying Traveling Jacks. Begin by doing stationary Jumping Jacks for approximately three seconds. As you continue, slowly move forward while your feet and arms maintain the Jumping Jack pattern. Move 5 to 10 yards and then briefly rest. To further challenge and stimulate the body, return to the starting point by doing backward Traveling Jacks. In general, Traveling Jacks lend themselves to a quicker tempo and smaller moves than in-place Jumping Jacks. Although the tempo of the arm and the legs is quicker with Traveling Jacks, the rate at which you cover ground should be slow.

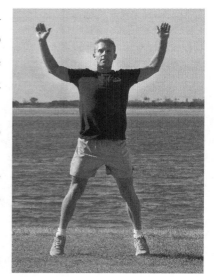

Traveling Jacks can also be done laterally. Begin with stationary Jumping Jacks and then cover ground to the left while continuing to jump the feet and swing the arms out and in. Then reverse direction to the right.

The Traveling Jack series is a more dynamic, neurologically stimulating and sports-specific activity for athletes whose games require multi-directional movements. By progressing from small stationary Jumping Jacks to larger stationary Jumping Jacks and then on to quicker Traveling Jacks, the body moves from low stimulation to a more game-ready higher stimulation, thus better preparing the body for the reactive demands of the sport.

PROGRAM DESIGN FOR JUMPING JACKS

- 4 sets of stationary Jumping Jacks approximately 30 seconds in length, or
- 6 sets of Traveling Jacks approximately 20 seconds in length and 10 yards in distance (2 repetitions each of Forward, Backward and Lateral Jacks)
- Rest 10 seconds between sets

Warm-Up Element Two: Dynamic Stretching

Support for a more dynamic warm up (DWU) has grown in recent years, because several investigations have shown the potential for acute, static stretching to degrade performance on vertical jumps, short sprints, tasks requiring maximal voluntary contractions, muscle strength-endurance performance, balance challenges, and reaction time.

—Danny J. McMillian et al., "Dynamic vs. Static-Stretching Warm Up: The Effect on Power and Agility Performance", *Journal of Strength and Conditioning Research*, 2006, 20(3), 492—499

Dynamic stretching is an activity that takes the body through sport-specific movements and general range-of-motion patterns from low to gradually increasing intensity levels. The purpose of dynamic stretching is to activate muscles, stimulate the nervous system and prepare the body and mind for the specific demands of a sport. This preparation systematically takes the body through movement patterns that collectively replicate the primary movements of that sport. These movements go from relatively small range-of-motion patterns and intensity to increasingly larger and more rigorous patterns. Scientific research overwhelmingly demonstrates the superiority of dynamic stretching compared to static stretching as a vehicle to safely improve general preparedness prior to a workout or a competition. Some dynamic stretches, such as those that focus on major muscle groups in the body, are beneficial for all athletic activities. Other dynamic stretches, such as rotational stretching, are more targeted and beneficial for particular athletic activities, such as swimming and kayaking, which involve repeated rotational movement.

It is your responsibility as an athlete to identify the specific demands of your sport. In doing so, you will be better able to prepare for individual training sessions or competition. In addition, by adding one or two dynamic stretches that are unlike the demands and movements of your sport, you provide much-needed flexibility and countermovement to the smaller and often subordinate muscles involved in your sport. This has a balancing effect on the body.

Dynamic stretching not only increases neurological functioning, mobility and mental preparedness, but also serves as a tool to assess your body's relative level of readiness. By being attentive to aches, pains, and your relative comfort level during dynamic stretching, you will be better prepared to make decisions about the intensity and duration of a workout session. Armed with such information, you can substitute, add, or delete aspects of your workout routine to minimize unnecessary wear and tear. Such mindfulness, combined with judicious choices based on the information you assimilate during this early phase of your workout, are at the heart of *Going the Distance*. Over time, such attention will help you bypass injuries and the interruptions they cause in training cycles.

Proper Posture/Starting Position for Most Dynamic Stretches

- Feet hip-width apart
- Knees slightly bent
- Hips in vertical alignment with heels
- Pelvis neutral, not tipped forward or backwards, throughout
- Long extended torso
- Chest broad
- Shoulders relaxed, down, and slightly pulled back
- Chin neutral
- Facial muscles relaxed
- Crown of the head high towards the sky (vertical polarity)

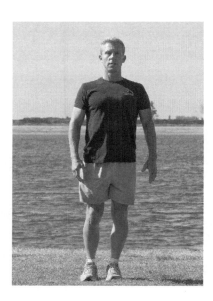

PROGRAM DESIGN FOR EACH OF THE DYNAMIC STRETCHES

• 2 sets of 20 seconds of each of the stretches listed below

• All dynamic stretches can be done in place or while moving

In general, the progression should go from an in-place position to forward-moving, then to backward-moving and lastly to lateral- and diagonally-moving patterns. Beginners would benefit from initially doing the stretches in place, preferably in front of a mirror to get visual feedback.

Form Walking

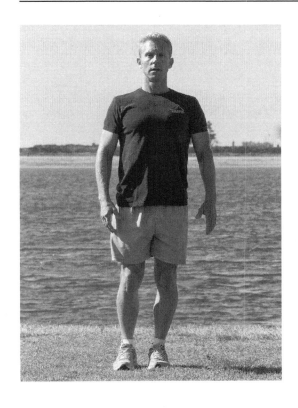
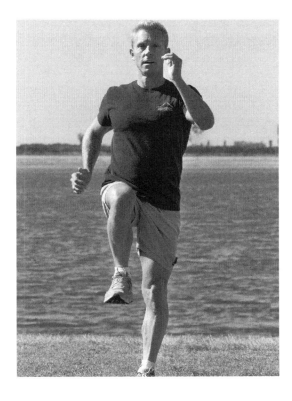

- Take one step forward and lift your right knee to hip height, keeping your right foot parallel to the ground. Avoid leaning forward or back.
- As the right leg rises up, slowly lift the left arm in a slow running motion.
- Slowly lower right knee and left arm back to starting position.
- Repeat the pattern on the opposite side.

Knee Tucks

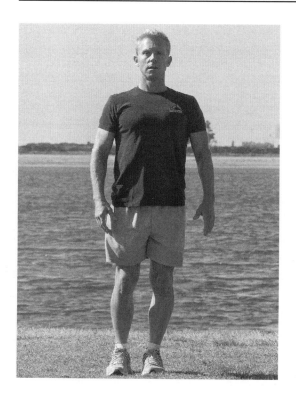 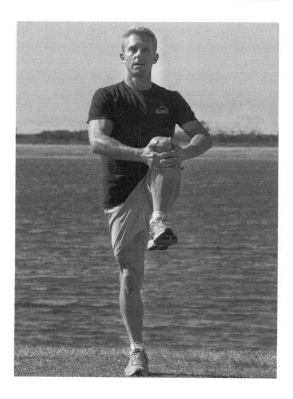

- Using primarily the muscles of the front of the thigh, lift the left knee as high as possible.
- At the top the movement, use both hands to gently bring the knee up slightly higher.
- Slowly lower the leg and then repeat on the other side.

Reverse Lunges

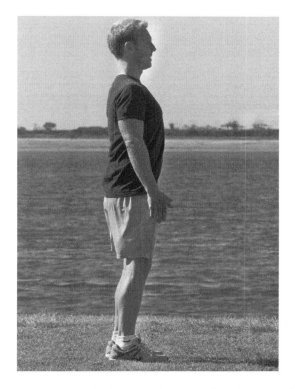 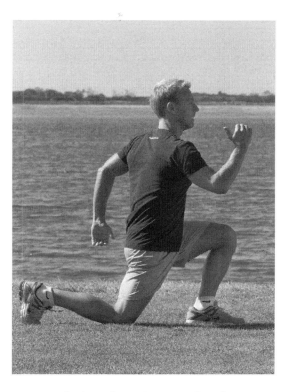

For more information and advanced options go to GoingtheDistancebook.com/ coaching-tips/ and choose Reverse Lunge.

- Step your right leg BACK about 1 to 3 feet, gently landing on the ball of the foot.
- As the back foot lands, bend both the back knee and the front knee, lowering your body into a lunge position. The front knee should start and remain on top of the front heel, not on top of or in front of the toes.
- Step the trail leg forward to return to the starting position. Repeat on the other side.

I suggest only going halfway down when initially executing this dynamic stretch. As balance, flexibility, and coordination improve, you can progress into a full reverse lunge with the back knee gently touching the ground. For advanced athletes, a side bend and torso twist can be added to the reverse lunge to better replicate the demands of certain sports. A forward lunge can be substituted for the reverse lunge for athletes with sufficient strength and balance.

Tick Tocks

Tick Tocks are old-fashioned side bends done slowly but continuously, as opposed to going to one side and holding the stretch statically.

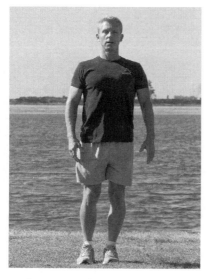 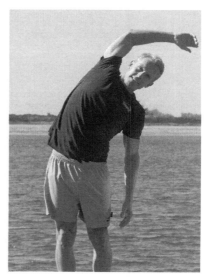

- From the starting position, slowly bend your torso to the left and bring your right arm up and over the body to a side-bending position.
- Return towards the center without stopping and bend to the right side, bringing the left arm up and over while bending to the right.

14

- Allow the elbow in the top arm to bend, adding further stretch to the arm. This stretch is most beneficial when done in place by all ability levels.

Soldiers

Soldiers resemble an exaggerated version of many military marches.

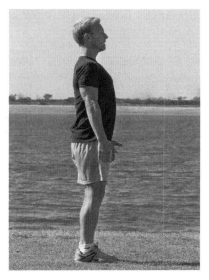 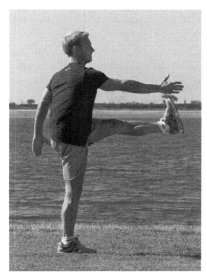

- From the starting position, lift the left leg as high as possible, straight out in front of you with minimal bend in the knee.
- Raise the opposite arm of the leg that is moving up in front of your body.
- Repeat this movement with the opposite leg and arm. Toes can be flexed back when the leg is at maximum height to increase the stretch in the calf.

External Hip Rotation

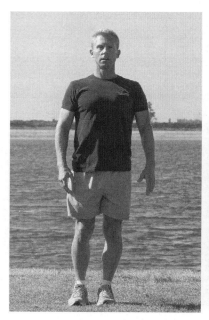 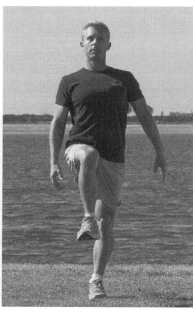 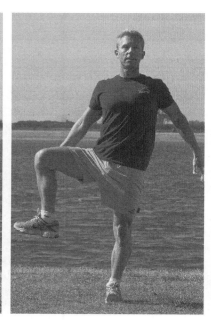

- From the starting position, lift the right knee up in front of the body and attempt to maintain a 90° angle in that knee. Keep the bottom of the lifted foot parallel to the ground.
- Rotate the lifted knee out and back to the outside while keeping the angle at the pelvis and the knee unchanged.
- Slowly lower the leg and the foot back to the starting position and repeat with the other leg. Continue to alternate legs.

The Skier

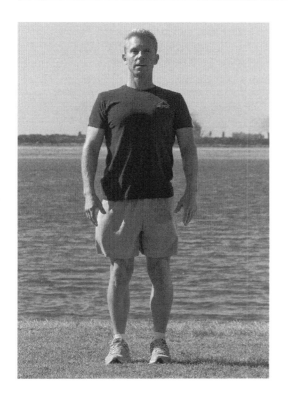 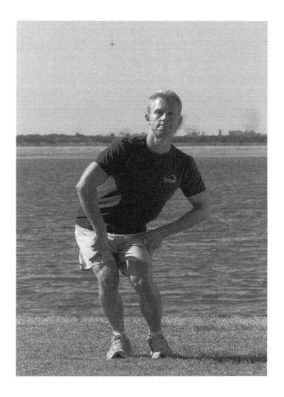

- From the starting position, hinge your hips slightly back as you slowly bend both knees to the right.
- Shift your weight to the right outer hip, putting moderate pressure into the right hip and the upper right thigh.
- Stand back up to the starting position, and without resting, bend both knees and shift your weight to the left, putting pressure into the left hip and the outer left thigh. Repeat.

Sumo Squats

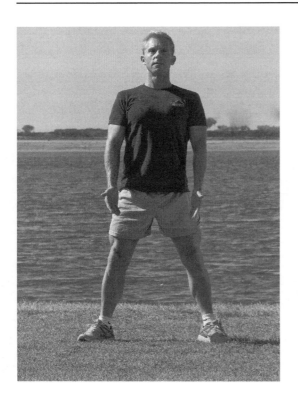 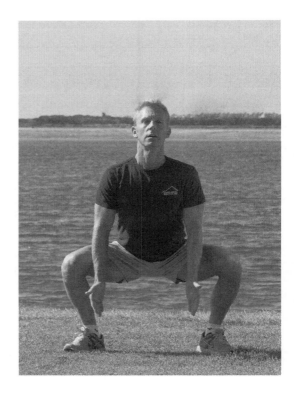

- Start with your feet shoulder-width apart, toes pointing slightly outward. Slowly bend both knees, dropping your hips back and down, lowering into a half knee-bend squatting position.
- Keep chest up, chin neutral and lower back mostly flat, allowing only for the natural curve of the spine, as you press weight evenly into your midfoot and heels to rise back up into the starting position.
- Keep your knees over your heels, and keep your knees in alignment with the toes at all times. Repeat.

Lateral Knee Bends

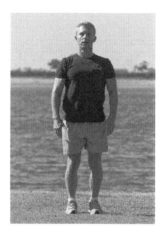 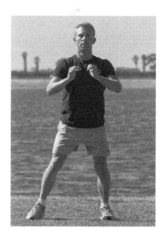

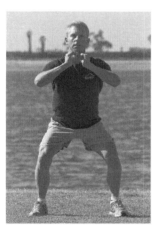 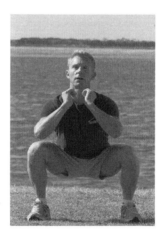

- From the starting position, step your right leg farther out to the side 6 to 12 inches. As your right foot contacts the ground, slowly lower the body into a half-knee bend (a squat).
- Press your weight evenly into the mid-foot and heel of both feet and press up and back into the original starting position in one fluid move.
- Repeat and then switch sides.
- Keep your knees on top of your heels and in alignment with your toes at all times.

Warm-Up Element Three: Progressive Sport-Specific Movement

As previously mentioned, the most important aspect of any warm-up is the gradual progression from lower to higher levels of intensity. If all you do is start slow and gradually build intensity in your actual sport, you will be doing your body a significant service as opposed to jumping right in and playing hard right away; unfortunately, as athletes we do not tend to defer our competitiveness for the sake of a proper warm-up. That said, for those wishing to make maximum gains in performance and maximize their athletic longevity, the final element of a warm-up should include movements, intervals and energy bursts similar to those you will experience during your practice or in your competition. For example, when preparing to play basketball, warm-up progression should move from a jog up and down the court to a jog with intervals of short bursts of speed. These intervals should be done at increasingly higher levels of intensity and should eventually include high-speed, lateral movements and change-of-direction drills. For fitness enthusiasts that typically walk, jog, hike, or do exclusively low-intensity aerobic exercise, this aspect will not be as necessary. The fitness enthusiast would be well-served at this point to include some low-intensity but varied moves, such as a hiker walking or jogging backwards on safe terrain or a swimmer cycling through different strokes other than her primary stroke of choice, for balanced strength development.

At first glance, such an extensive approach to warming up may seem excessive, and can seem like an obstacle that negatively affects the total time available for playing the actual sport. In the short run, this may be true. However, over time, such an approach will be a key component to a formula that potentially adds years to your playing life and improves the quality of your play. Also, keep in mind that a personalized and abbreviated selection of dynamic stretches still has great value if you take the time to choose the ones most relevant to your activity.

A sequence of dynamic exercises that utilizes the full range of joint mobility can prepare the body for the more intensive activities without prior static stretching, especially if such movements are initially performed slowly and smoothly during the warm-up.

—Rheba E. Vetter, "Effects of Six Warm-Up Protocols on Sprint and Jump Performance," *Journal of Strength and Conditioning Research*, 2007, 21(3), 819—823

Versions of this warm-up format are being taught at rehab centers, colleges and professional training rooms across the country. Leading fitness institutions such as the National Strength and Conditioning Association, the American Council on Exercise, and the American College of Sports Medicine have also endorsed this type of warm-up format. The most recent scientific research, as well as my practical experience competing and winning at the national and international levels, further supports the profound value of a targeted, progressive and extensive warm-up process. I strongly urge you to view the warm-up process as part of the entire workout and not separate from the training session or competition itself. Many athletes, especially older athletes, spend little or no time on this critical element of training and unknowingly lose an opportunity to bridge the gap to optimum performance. If you are seriously committed to going the distance, warming up is a crucial first step. If you can change the way you think about warming up and make small improvements to your current routine, you will see tangible results in the quality of your training, competing and recreation for many years to come.

Chapter Two:
Core Stability and Major Joint Stability

Functional stability is paramount to lifelong good health and injury prevention. Having good positional awareness and stability provides an important platform upon which strength can be built and allows us to move more efficiently during our daily activities. Whether you're an older adult who is looking to prevent injury or a young athlete who wants to improve his or her ability, optimal stability can lead to both an improved quality of life and enhanced athletic performance.

—Stewart Sanders, DPT, ATC,
Owner - Golf Performance Clinic, Physical Therapist - Sharp Rees-Stealy

Core Stability (CS)—that is, stability of the middle third of the body—and Major Joint Stability (MJS) training are perhaps the two most important components for developing and maintaining a functional, durable and resilient body for life. My approach to core stability focuses on training the major and important minor muscles of the middle part of the body, from the upper thigh through the mid-back. MJS includes training both large and small muscle groups that are critical to the integrity of key joints that affect mobility and athletic function. Although the physical demands of all sports are different, across most sports the major joints in the body are exposed to both the stress of repetitive movements and high-intensity loads, both of which can lead to serious injury. The shoulders for swimmers, the knees for runners and the lower back for golfers are examples of major joints that affect form, function and athletic longevity.

Intelligent and consistent attention to CS and MJS training in your exercise routine significantly decreases the likelihood of injury. Although prime movers (major muscles) of both the core and important load-bearing joints require specific training to maximize function, much of stability training concentrates on strengthening small antagonist (opposing) and synergist (enhancing) muscles that augment and balance the often stronger and larger prime movers. This deliberate approach to balancing strength across a joint adds functional integrity to the joint. Even accomplished and well-trained athletes often overlook these smaller, less familiar muscles, which are so essential to long-term participation in a sport.

Core stability has received a tremendous amount of media attention in the last decade, particularly in fitness magazines and through advertisements for health clubs. But few recreational athletes, and even many coaches and trainers, sufficiently understand the specific muscle groups that need attention and do not make training these muscles a priority. Many health clubs promote core stability through a variety of group fitness classes, which often focus only on abdominal crunching, knee lifting or aggressive plyometric exercises. Although the intention is good, and many of the exercises have value for certain populations, these exercises often put excessive strain on the body and expose athletes—especially older athletes—to unnecessary risk of injury. Commonly, little to no attention is paid to proper difficulty progression, and many participants attempt to execute high intensity exercises that compromise the integrity of their lower backs, especially when done in hourlong classes.

Regular, targeted training of the core and major joints not only decreases the likelihood of injury, but can also lead directly to performance improvement through improved force production and improved neurological function. The middle body is a key source of power for many athletic movements. In particular, golfers, swimmers and tennis players should recognize that their power comes from this area. Effectively transferring energy from the middle body out to the extremities determines, to a large extent, how far a golfer can hit a golf ball, how well a swimmer can improve her turns and starts, and how well a tennis player can transfer energy from his racket to the ball.

CST and MJS training can be done efficiently during the warm-up or the cool-down phases of your workout. When done as part of a warm-up, the relatively low impact of these exercises is a forgiving way to gradually increase intensity and focus. When done as part of a cool-down, these exercises will assist the body in gradually calming and lowering heart rate, respiration, and athletic excitation. The lower back, knees and shoulders are arguably the three most important and most vulnerable joints, subject to wear and tear and acute trauma across most sports, and will therefore be the focus of my discussion.

The exercises that follow are categorized under their primary area of benefit. However, almost all of them are multi-joint exercises and serve as stabilizers for multiple joints in the kinetic chain. Similarly, any movement done with awareness and some amount of recruitment (that is, lifting up or gently tightening in of the abdomen) can have real strengthening value for the middle body. The exercises below should be done in a progression from low to high intensity and from a relatively low volume (number of sets and repetitions) to a higher volume. If you experience any acute irritation while performing these exercises, stop and consult a physician to determine an appropriate path for CS and MJS.

PROGRAM DESIGN FOR ALL STABILITY EXERCISES

- **Two to three sets of 10 repetitions**

- **Rest 15 seconds between sets if doing all sets of one exercise at a time.**

- **Little to no rest is required if alternating exercises and contrasting body parts.**

Advanced Options

- For each of the exercises listed below, instability tools (rollers, balls, pads, disks, bands, etc.) can be used to make the exercise more difficult.
- Beginners and those recovering from an injury should start on the ground without any added instability devices and focus on pain-free movement.

Waterman Series

The Waterman Series consists of three exercises which can be done on the ground or on a physioball. Although the series is especially targeted for aquatic athletes, requiring posterior body endurance, it is beneficial for developing core stability for all land-based athletes as well. The primary muscles engaged are the lumbar spine stabilizers, hamstrings, hip rotators and extensors, back extensors, and shoulder flexors.

Proper Posture and Starting Position for Waterman Exercises

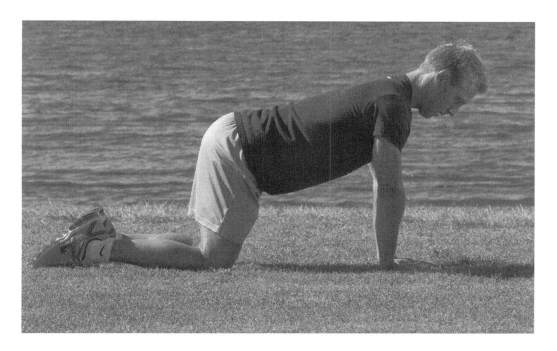

- All-fours position
- Hands under shoulders, knees under hips
- Back flat, pelvis neutral, eyes looking down throughout

Super Heroes

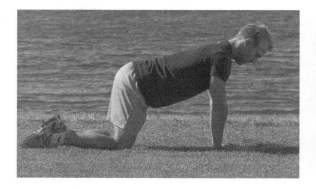 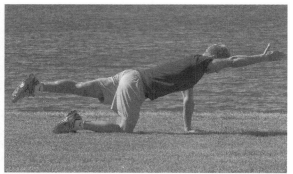

- Slowly extend your right arm forward and up to shoulder height, while at the same time extending left leg back and up to hip height.
- Pause and slowly lower arm and leg back to starting position and repeat.

Flying Super Heroes

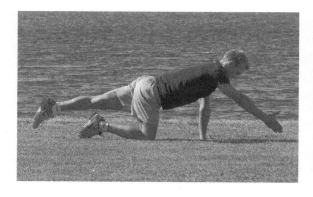 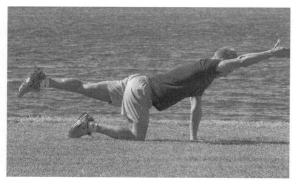

- Slowly extend your right arm up to shoulder height, while at the same time slowly extending the left leg back and up to hip height.

28

- Pause. Without bending the right elbow and the left knee, slowly lower arm and leg until fingertips and toes touch the ground.
- Repeat and continue movement, keeping elbow and knee straight throughout.

Wonder Dogs

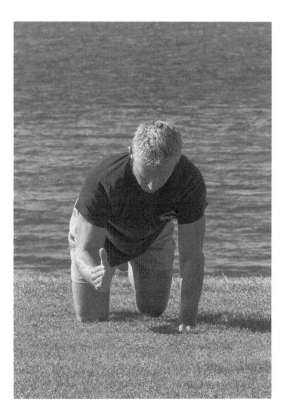 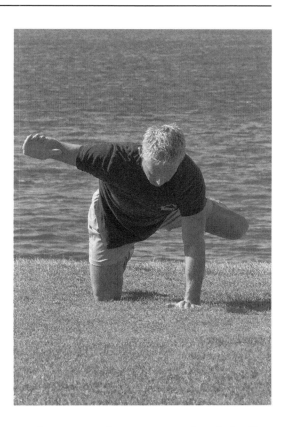

Note: This Waterman exercise should be done on the ground, not on a physioball.

- Slowly raise your right arm up and out to the side, keeping your elbow at a 90° angle while at the same time raising your left knee up and out to hip height.
- Pause and slowly lower arm and leg back to starting position and repeat.

Basic Bridge

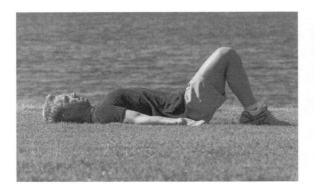 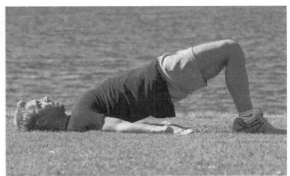

- Lie on your back with both knees bent, feet parallel and firmly into the ground.
- Keep your torso and neck long and shoulders broad.
- Press your weight evenly into both feet and then raise the lower, middle and upper back off the ground.
- Pause when the thighs, hips and chest are in one parallel plane. Avoid putting excess weight into the neck area. Instead, spread the weight broadly across the shoulders.
- Slowly lower the upper, middle and then finally the lower back into the ground and repeat without resting.

Pelvic Tilts

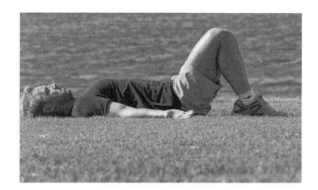 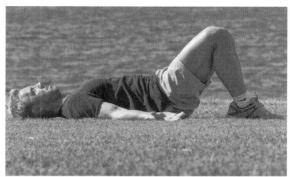

- Lie on the ground on your back, knees bent, thighs parallel and feet planted firmly and evenly on the ground.
- Keep your entire torso and neck long, shoulders broad, head resting on the ground.
- Inhale to prepare, and then firmly press your lower back into the ground by contracting the lower abdominal muscles while slowly exhaling.
- Hold lower abdominal contraction for three seconds, inhale slowly as you relax your abdominal muscles, and return to starting position.
- Repeat without resting.

Single Leg, Modified Leg Lifts

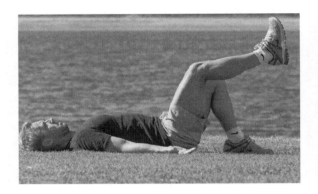 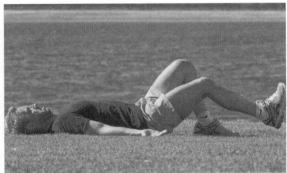

- Lie on the ground on your back with left knee bent and left foot firmly and evenly on the ground.
- Start your right foot off the ground, right knee bent at a 90° angle, thighs parallel.
- Keep your entire torso and neck long, shoulders broad, head resting on the ground.
- Keep left knee at a 90° angle throughout.
- Firmly press your lower back into the ground, assuming the pelvic tilt position.
- While maintaining the pelvic tilt position, slowly lower your right heel down and away from the body, and stop as the right heel gently touches the ground.
- Raise your right knee slowly back to starting position.
- Repeat and switch legs.
- Remember to hold the pelvic tilt throughout the entire exercise.

Classic Crunches

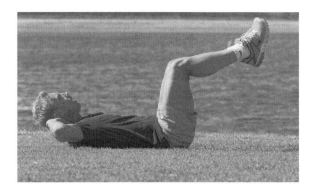 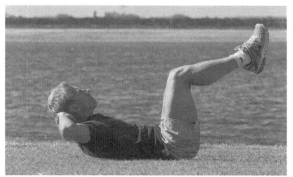

- Lie on the ground on your back, with your hands interlocked behind your head (across your chest if you have neck problems). Your shoulder blades should be just barely off the ground.
- Feet are off the ground and knees are bent at a 90° angle.
- Inhale to prepare and exhale as you slowly raise your chest up towards the sky, keeping elbows wide, with neck in a relaxed, neutral position, supported in your hands.
- Pause at maximum height and slowly lower back to starting position. Repeat without resting.

Back Extensions

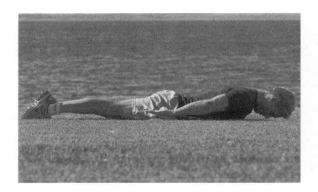 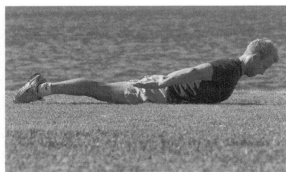

- Lie face-down with legs and feet resting on the ground, eyes looking down, nose just barely off the ground.
- Keep your hands by your side, about an inch off the ground, with palms facing up.
- Inhale to prepare and exhale as you slowly engage the muscles of the lower, middle and upper back to raise your torso up.
- Pause at near-maximum height, eyes still gazing down, neck long and relaxed. Make sure your feet stay down throughout the exercise.
- Slowly lower back to starting position and repeat without resting.

Plank

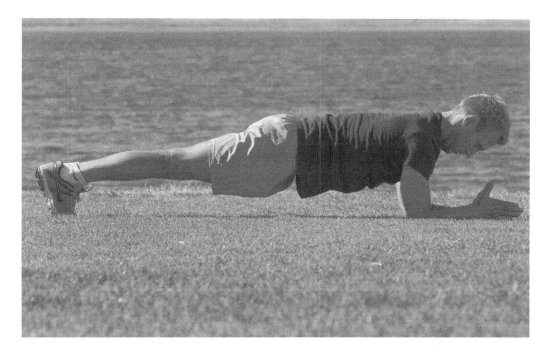

- Lie face-down with only your elbows and toes on the ground.
- Elbows should be aligned under the shoulders, neck should be long, eyes looking down at the mat.
- Keep your entire spine, from lower back to neck, in alignment, and keep your lower back flat throughout the entire exercise.
- Hold for approximately 10 to 20 seconds. This constitutes one set.
- Breathe slowly and steadily; do not hold your breath.

Side Plank

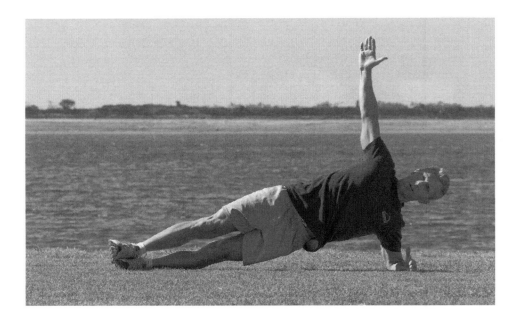

- Lie on your side with only your left elbow, forearm, and feet touching the ground.
- Left elbow should be lined up underneath the left shoulder. Your entire spine should be in alignment.
- Hold for 20 seconds. Avoid twisting or dropping your torso. Rest and repeat on the other side. 20 seconds on each side constitutes one set.
- Breathe slowly and steadily. Do not hold your breath.

Knee Stability Exercises

All of the knee stability exercises can be done using only your body weight as resistance. That said, the body gets stronger in response to gradual increases in load. Dumbbells, barbells and sandbags are very good external tools to increase the intensity of knee-stabilizing exercises.

Single Leg Step-Ups

This exercise can be done using a step ranging from 1 inch to approximately 18 inches high, depending on your height, the relative health of your knees, and your athletic goals. The average person using this exercise for injury prevention should use a 6-inch step to start and gradually increase the height over time.

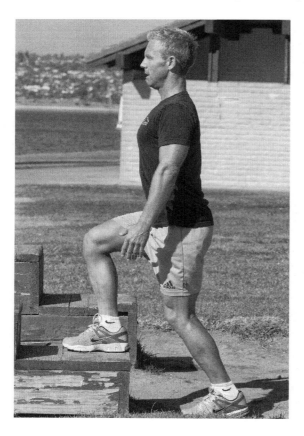 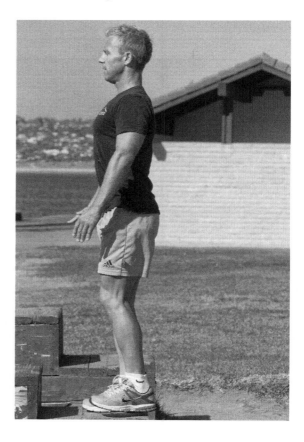

- To start, place your entire right foot firmly and evenly on the step. Keep your right knee over your right ankle throughout the entire exercise.

- Distribute your weight evenly onto both feet in the starting position.
- Firmly press most of your weight into the mid-foot and heel of your right foot as you step up and place your left foot up and onto the step.
- Slowly lower your left foot back to the starting position while keeping your right knee lined up over the right heel, without moving forward or collapsing inward.
- Repeat without resting. Switch legs.

Life Lifts

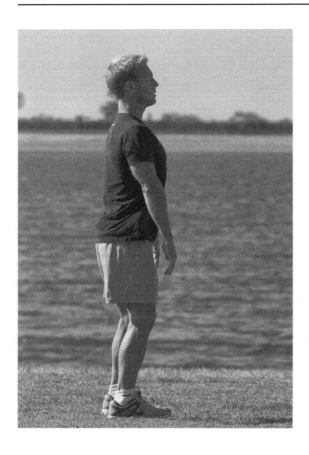 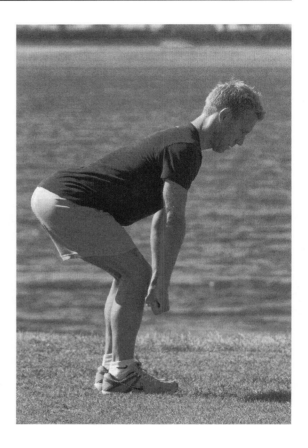

- Start with feet parallel and hip-width apart, weight primarily on mid-feet and heels, knees slightly bent, neck and torso long, chest broad, chin neutral.
- Slowly move your hips back in a hinging move.
- Keep your lower back flat and chest up as you bend your body forward.
- Slowly extend knees, hips, and back to return to the starting position
- Repeat without resting.

Reverse Lunges

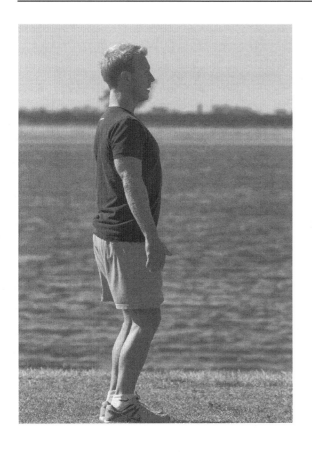 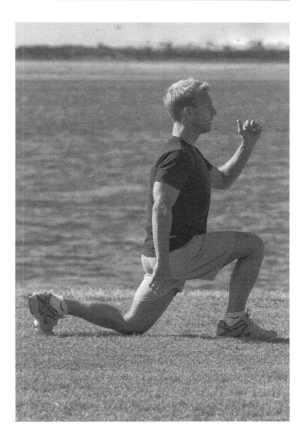

- Start with feet parallel and hip-width apart, knees slightly bent, neck and torso long, chest broad, chin neutral.
- Inhale as you step your left foot back approximately 18 to 36 inches, bending both knees and gently landing on the ball of your left foot.
- Exhale as you firmly press your weight onto your right foot to return to the starting position.
- Keep the right knee above the right ankle throughout the entire exercise. Keep your torso long and chest up throughout.
- Alternate sides each repetition.

Lateral Knee Bends

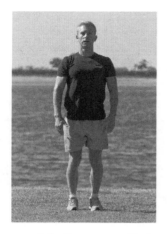 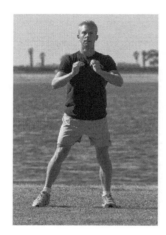

- Start with feet parallel and hip-width apart, knees slightly bent, neck and torso long, chest broad, chin neutral.
- Step your right foot out to the right 6 to 18 inches.

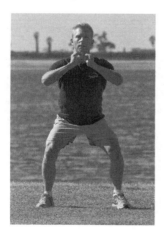 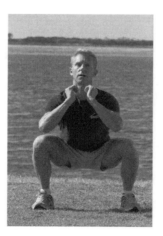

- As the right foot makes contact with the ground, slowly lower into squat position.
- Point your toes forward or slightly outward throughout the exercise.

- Keep your knees over your ankles without collapsing inward or moving forward in front of the toes.
- Press your weight evenly into both feet to rise up out of the squat and back into the starting position.
- Repeat without resting. Repeat on the left side.

Clam Shell

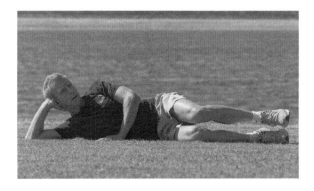 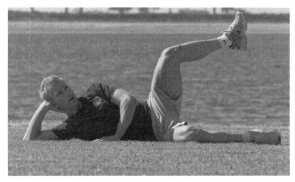

Ankle weights or tubing can be good additional forms of resistance for this exercise.

- Lie on your right side with your right hand or arm supporting your neck.
- Knees should be one on top of the other, off to the right at a 90° angle.
- Inhale to prepare. Exhale as you raise your left knee and hip up and out to near-maximum height.
- Pause and slowly inhale as you lower your left knee back to the starting position. Repeat without resting. Switch sides.
- Pelvis and torso should be still and abdominal muscles should remain engaged throughout.

Shoulder Stability Exercises

Shoulder stability exercises can be executed using dumbbells, resistance tubing, or a cable machine. The tools I've chosen to illustrate the exercises are, in my opinion, the best for each exercise.

External Rotation

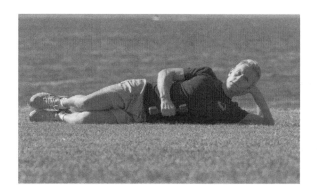 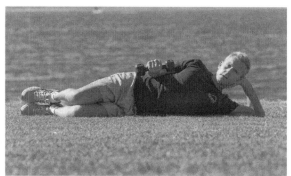

- Lie on your left side with your left hand or arm supporting your neck, with shoulder blades pulled back and gently tucked in and down.
- Grasp the dumbbell with your right hand. Your right arm should be flat across your body.
- Keep your elbow back at your side, bent at a 90° angle.
- Exhale as you slowly rotate your lower arm away from your body without turning your body, breaking the flat angle of your right wrist, or allowing your elbow to come off the side of your body.
- Inhale as you very slowly rotate the dumbbell across your body to the starting position.
- Keep shoulder blades back and down throughout.
- Repeat and then switch sides.

External Rotation with arm raised to 90°

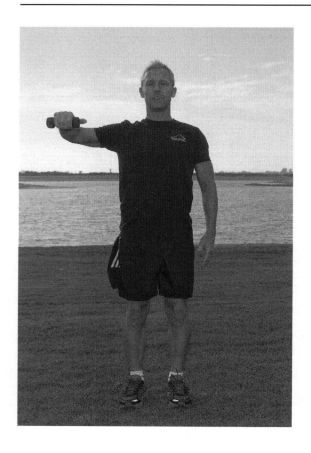 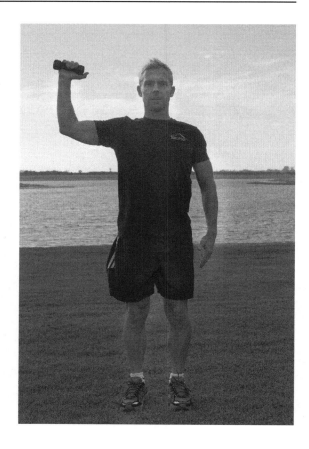

- Stand tall, with your feet hip-width apart and shoulder blades pulled back and gently tucked in and down.
- Raise your right arm to shoulder height, with the elbow bent at a 90° angle, and grasp dumbbell with palm facing down.
- Keep upper arm even with shoulder as you rotate lower arm to near maximum height, ending with palm facing away.
- Repeat on other side.

Note: Do not move shoulder blades during this exercise.

Serratus Reach: "The Boxer"

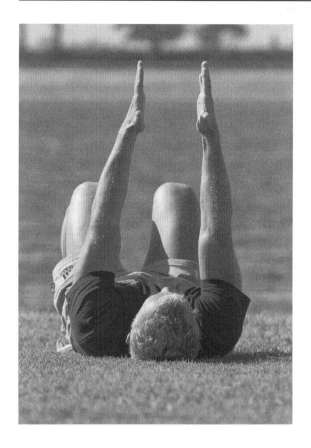 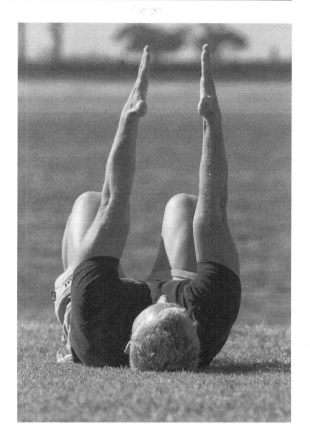

- Lie on your back, either on the ground or on a Styrofoam roller or physioball, with knees bent and parallel, feet firmly planted into the ground.
- Keep your neck and torso long, shoulders broad, and head resting on the ground, both arms extended towards the sky.
- Inhale to prepare. As you exhale, reach your hands as high as possible towards the sky without moving your torso or neck off the ground.
- Keep your elbows straight throughout the entire exercise.

- Pause in the arms extended position, then slowly lower your arms back down into the starting position. Repeat.
- To better hit the entire Serratus Anterior, one set can done as described above, a second set can be done with your arms moving slightly back, and a third set with your arms moving slightly forward.

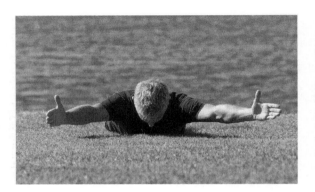 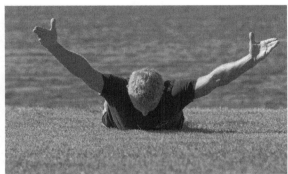

Y-Pattern

- Lie face down on the ground, on a bench or on a physioball, eyes gazing downward, with your neck long.
- Hold your arms in front of your body, elbows locked, thumbs pointing upward, creating a Y shape with your torso and arms.
- Inhale to prepare. Exhale as you slowly lift your extended arms off the ground to near-maximum height.
- Pause in the extended Y position, then slowly lower arms back to starting position.
- Keep torso long and still throughout the entire exercise, back extensor muscles active but not hyperextended, and maintain the Y position throughout.
- Repeat without resting.

- Shoulder blades should remain down and slightly drawn in throughout the entire exercise. You may need to reset them between reps.

T-Pattern

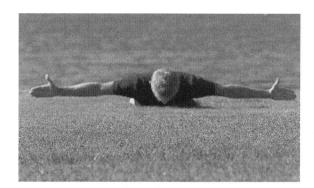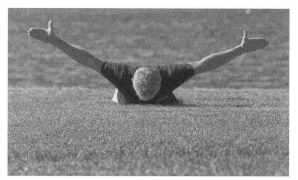

- Lie face down on the ground, on a bench or on a physio-ball, eyes gazing downward, with your neck long.
- Hold your arms out to the side, elbows locked, thumbs pointing upward, creating a T shape with your torso and arms.
- Inhale to prepare. Exhale as you slowly lift your extended arms off the ground to near-maximum height.
- Pause in the extended T position, then slowly lower arms back to starting position.
- Keep torso long and still throughout the entire exercise, with back extensor muscles active but not hyperextended, and maintain the T position throughout.
- Repeat without resting.
- Shoulder blades should remain down and slightly drawn in.

I-Pattern

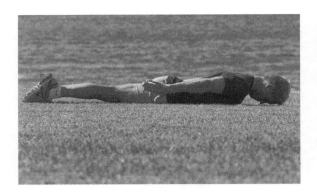 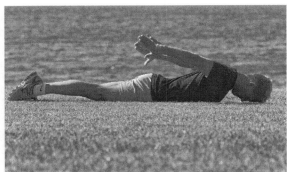

- Lie face down on the ground, on a bench or on a physioball, eyes gazing downward, with your neck long.
- Hold your arms by your sides, elbows locked, thumbs pointing downward, creating an I shape with your torso and arms.
- Inhale to prepare. Exhale as you slowly lift your extended arms off the ground to near-maximum height, drawing the shoulder blades in and slightly down.
- Pause in the extended I position, and then slowly lower arms back to starting position.
- Keep torso long and still throughout the entire exercise, back extensor muscles active but not hyperextended, and maintain the I position throughout.
- Repeat without resting.
- Shoulder blades should remain down and slightly drawn in throughout the entire exercise.

The CS and MJS exercises included above represent a sound starting point for implementing a well-rounded stability routine. Depending on the particular physical demands of your sport, focus on those exercises that most support the primary movement patterns of that sport. For example, it would be wise for a cyclist to focus significantly on stabilizing and strengthening the extensor muscles of the back by doing the Waterman Series and back extensions, as those endurance muscles are largely responsible for the cyclist's ability to remain comfortable in the forward-leaning position of cycling. The cyclist would also do well to include some of the shoulder stability exercises, as stability and posterior shoulder strength is key to maintaining good posture on and off the bike. Less stability attention would be required of the knee, as cycling itself puts quite a well-balanced load on the front and back of the legs.

A swimmer or a surfer would be well-served by focusing on shoulder stability exercises, as the repetitive motions of their sport put the shoulders at great risk of injury.

All of the exercises above can be manipulated to increase or decrease relative intensity. As your technique improves, it is important to gradually increase the difficulty of the exercises, first by systematically adding more repetitions, sets, instability tools and resistance, and then by eventually adding more advanced versions. Remember that the body only changes if it is stressed beyond its current capability level. If done gradually through increased volume, load and instability tools, you will feel a tangible improvement in strength and sturdiness and likely an improved economy of movement in your sport.

Chapter Three:
Cool-Down

I have consistently found that an emphasis on proper recovery at the end of work-outs has been an effective way to promote both better performance and injury prevention. The keys are using that time to cool the body down slowly, promote flexibility, and address any issues that might be present at the time or have been historical problems for the athlete, and refuel the system. Achieving these through a comprehensive and regimented process usually leads to greatest success, as each plays a critical role in recovery, regeneration, and injury prevention.

—Mick Gieskes, Sprint Coach, University of California
San Diego Track & Field and Masters Coach Movin Shoes Running Centers

The primary way to include my Third Pillar of Lifelong Fitness, Recovery, is to regularly execute a proper cool-down after all workouts. A thorough cool-down is an essential tool for increasing flexibility as well as initiating and speeding up recovery. In addition, a complete and balanced cool-down indirectly improves performance and directly minimizes the risk of overuse injuries. Failure to deliberately cool, restore, and reset the body after even moderate-intensity exercise not only limits potential athletic gains but also significantly increases the likelihood of injuries. Due to time constraints and lack of awareness of their importance, cool-downs are commonly omitted from training routines.

I believe no other element contributes as significantly or directly to long-term athletic performance and longevity than regular execution of a thorough cool-down. Research and my decades of competing and coaching further confirm the importance of recovery. As Phillip A. Bishop, Eric Jones and A. Krista Woods note in their article "Recovery from Training: A Brief Review," "Even the most dedicated athlete spends much more time in recovery than in active training... Recovery from training is one of the most important aspects of improving athletic performance" (*Journal of Strength and Conditioning Research*, 22(3), 1015—1024).

Like a proper warm-up, a cool-down has both physiological and psychological benefits. The physiological goals of a proper cool-down are to lower heart rate, blood pressure, respiration, and inflammatory responses. In addition, a cool-down helps leave body systems more relaxed and poised to reap the benefits of the workout.

Similarly, a deliberate cool-down has profound psychological and emotional benefits, serving as a calming and transitional episode from sports or training to everyday life. By taking time to cool-down after exercise, you will feel more grounded and better equipped to function and handle the challenges that await you. Like a proper warm-up, there are three sequential elements to a proper cool-down which aid in increasing flexibility, repairing tissue and initiating a full recovery:

- General aerobic cool-down
- Static stretching
- Orthopedic self-care

General Aerobic Cool-Down

A general aerobic cool-down involves a deliberate lowering of intensity in the final portion of a workout and lasts for about five to fifteen minutes. For example, when an athlete finishes a brisk thirty-minute run, he could transition into a walk or a jog at a significantly lower level of intensity for the final several minutes of the run. The same principle is true for a cyclist. After completing a road ride or a spin class, he would be well-served to ride his bike at a significantly lower level of exertion for several minutes before finishing the ride. That same cyclist would also benefit from continuing his cool-down off the bike with several minutes of low-intensity walking, jogging, or skipping, if the proper environment is available. The time spent by the cyclist on his feet and off of the saddle not only contributes to the basic goals of the cool-down, but also unloads muscles and joints from the relatively static position of cycling.

The higher the intensity of the workout, and the more orthopedic issues an athlete has, the greater the importance of a deliberate and lengthy aerobic cool-down. This aerobic flush quiets, cools, calms and begins the recovery process. Although it's understandable that the basketball player wants to get in as many games as possible in a playing session, and the competitive swimmer as many high-intensity intervals as possible during a workout, to keep the engine performing at top speed and then abruptly turn it off is physically damaging and counterproductive to the mind/body machine. Although some of us can get away with it occasionally, the athletes that continually walk away without cooling down after moderate- to high-intensity training lose the opportunity to more expeditiously initiate the recovery process. In endurance sports, regularly including an extended aerobic cool-down has the additional benefit of providing some low wear and tear mileage.

STABILITY TRAINING

As mentioned in Chapter 1, stability training is ideally done as part of a gradually progressive warm-up when the body is fresh in order to increase the success of recruiting the small muscles that are the target of this training. Because much of the focus in stability training is on small, easily fatigued muscles, training them when they are fresh will improve neural recruitment patterns and ensure better form. However, since stability training is such an important part of injury prevention, longevity and performance, it is far better to include low- to moderate-intensity stability training as a last part of a general aerobic cool-down, even if the muscles are moderately fatigued, than to omit it entirely. See Chapter 2 for specific options.

Static Stretching

Static stretching is a slow and deliberate attempt to lengthen and loosen muscles and muscle systems. It should be done carefully, without bouncing or any ballistic moves. Slow, steady and deliberate breathing further increases the physical benefits and relaxing effect of static stretching. In this way, many styles of yoga can be a valid way to approach the needs of static stretching outside of your regular workouts. Although there are many styles of yoga, each with its own emphasis, Hatha is a term that describes almost all versions of physical poses and is the most popular form of yoga practiced in America today. The majority of Hatha classes are simply a flowing series of static stretches. The recent surge in yoga participation demonstrates the appeal of this feel-good activity. Computer and television use and increased time spent driving have left many of us, even non-athletes, feeling more tight, stressed, and achy than the previous generation, which was often more involved in physical work. Static stretching helps negate the negative consequences of our 21st-century minimal-movement work model quite effectively.

The optimum time within a workout for static stretching is immediately following a general aerobic cool-down or immediately following orthopedic self-care. Research and thousands of firsthand interviews I've conducted show that static stretching is a vital part of the recovery process that helps minimize post-workout soreness. In certain sports, athletes can actually begin some static stretching during their aerobic cool-down. For example, a cyclist in a spin class can safely stretch most upper body parts while still engaging in low-level aerobic riding. However, in most cases, you will find that static stretching is best done in a comfortable area, such as on a mat or on grass, where you can relax and comfortably complete your routine. Unlike dynamic stretching, which focuses on broad movement patterns to initiate pre-workout readiness and mobility, static stretching aims to isolate specific muscle groups and thus is performed slowly, holding each stretch for thirty to sixty seconds depending on the body part. Although all sports and fitness activities stress and tighten the body differently, the muscle groups around the major joints in the body—shoulders, lower back, and knees—require attention from athletes engaged in virtually all sports. You would be well-served by identifying the prime movers and the major muscles in your sport and, at a minimum, address those muscle groups after every workout.

The list below is a summary of stretches I believe are hugely beneficial for all athletes and for anyone committed to lifelong fitness and feeling more comfortable inside their own body.

PROGRAM DESIGN FOR STATIC STRETCHING AND ORTHOPEDIC SELF-CARE TECHNIQUES

- 1 to 2 sets of each or more as dictated by your body's needs
- Hold stretches for 30 to sixty seconds.

Vertical Hanging

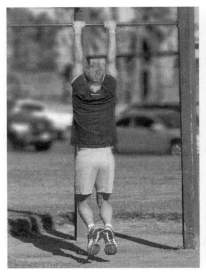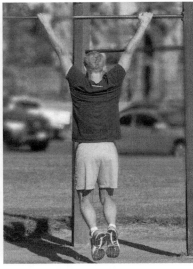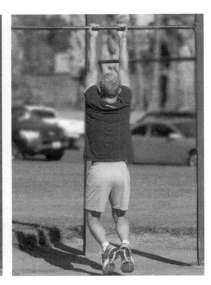

- Select a safe (non-moveable) device from which to hang.
- Vary hand grip position for each set of hangs, between narrow, wide, and reverse.
- Firmly hold the bar without excessive squeezing.
- Keep neck and spine long, in alignment and relaxed.
- It's ok if the feet touch the ground to help take some of the weight off of the hands.
- Focus on allowing the muscles along the sides, armpit area, and lower back to relax and lengthen.

Horizontal Hanging

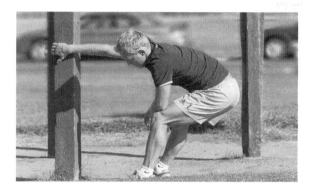 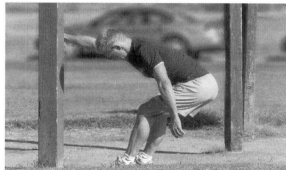

- Vary handgrip position by repetition from palms in to palms out.
- Firmly hold the bar without excessive squeezing.
- Use your legs and hips to help support much of your weight.
- Gently lean away, lengthening the tight segments from your armpits, along your outer rib cage, and down into your lower back.

Standing Side Bends

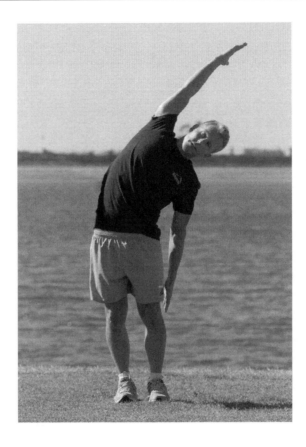

- Stand tall, with a slight bend in the knees, feet hip-width apart.
- Lift your torso, lengthen your abdomen, and gently draw in at the navel throughout.
- Slowly bend from the lower trunk to the left.
- Keep right arm in alignment with ear or head if your shoulder allows
- Stay open across the chest.
- Remember to keep breathing regular throughout.

Chest Opener

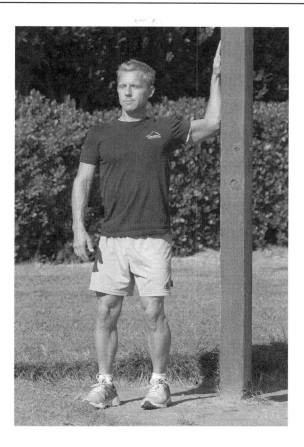

- Keep your chest up and shoulders broad.
- Hold your left elbow at shoulder height, palm facing in and gently pressing into a post or wall.
- Feet can be parallel or slightly offset.
- Maintain a flat, neutral lower back throughout.
- Use only light force into your left arm as you gently turn away, opening your body to the right.

Supported Lunge

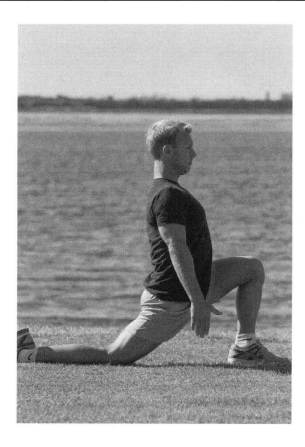

- Keep left knee aligned with ankle; do not allow it to bend past the ankle.
- Press right knee firmly into the ground and let the right hip open down towards the ground.
- Lift torso, gently drawing in abdomen throughout, and align entire spine.
- Keep your chest up and shoulders broad, with your shoulder blades gently drawn in and down throughout.
- Hold chin neutral (not tipped) and crown of the head high.

Pigeon

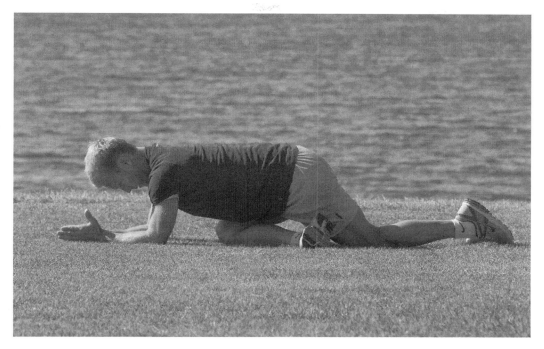

- Start in an all fours position, then bring right leg across center line at a relatively comfortable angle (there should be no pain in either knee).
- Keep elbows aligned under the shoulders, providing structural support.
- Maintain a long torso and neutral spine throughout.
- Keep your chest up and shoulders broad.
- Lengthen the back leg and extend toes.
- Pressure and stretch should be primarily in right outer hip. Avoid tipping or leaning.

Supine Hamstring

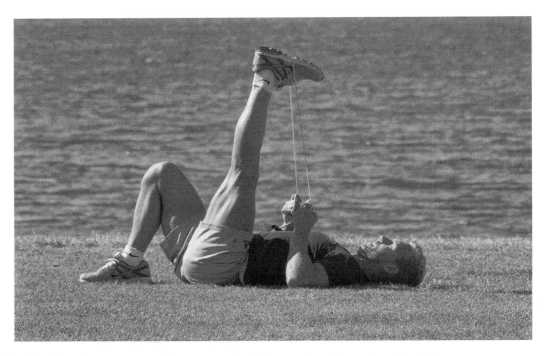

- Entire back rests on the ground with neck relaxed and chin slightly dropped.
- Bend right knee and place right foot into the ground for lower back support.
- Use a strap, band or towel to capture the left mid-foot.
- Keep the left knee slightly bent.
- Using as little force as necessary, pull the left leg up until the stretch is noticeable in the back of the left leg. Pause. Breathe regularly throughout, then gradually increase the stretch as the leg relaxes.
- Keep both hips flat on the ground throughout.

Alternate Leg Stretch

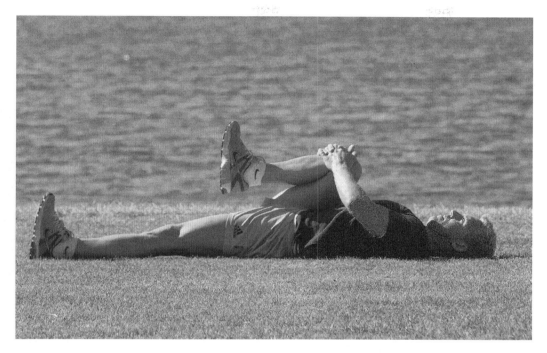

- Entire back rests on the ground with neck relaxed and chin slightly dropped.
- Gently grip the area just below the knee on the top of the right lower leg. Alternatively, you can also grip just above the knee on the back of the right leg.
- Draw the right leg up towards the abdomen and chest area, keeping the right knee in alignment with the right shoulder.
- Use as little force as possible to affect the stretch. Keep shoulders relaxed.
- Fully extend the left leg for a stretch across the hip crease, or bend the left leg for extra lower back support.

Spinal Twist

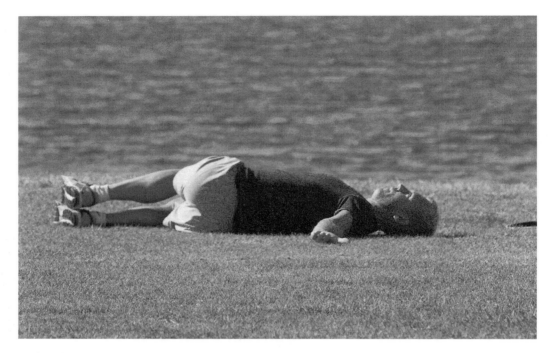

- Entire back rests on the ground with neck relaxed and chin slightly dropped.
- Keep shoulders broad and relaxed.
- Gently drop both knees over to the right without changing the angle of the spine or the shoulders. Much of the back will rise off the ground.
- A bolster can be place between the knees for additional support.
- Ideally, create and maintain right angles at the knees and hips, keeping both shoulders relaxed into the ground. Focus on gentle full breathing throughout entire stretch.

Orthopedic Self-Care

Orthopedic self-care (OSC) is a crucial element of peak performance and injury prevention and the last part of a proper cool-down. The goal of OSC is to systematically address parts of the body that are most vulnerable to injury or are already compromised by overuse or chronic injuries. Olympic and professional sports training rooms across the world dedicate significant space and attention to this critical aspect of recovery. From a very young age, I had the privilege of being exposed to athletic trainers and physical therapists who planted the seeds of awareness for this cool-down component. The time I spent working with a trainer at the Governor's Academy provided me my first exposure to the profound value of self-care modalities. Later on, plagued with overuse injuries in college, I once again learned ideas, techniques, methods and philosophies of healing and injury prevention through self-care. The certified athletic trainers at San Diego State University helped further advance my understanding of the necessity of self-care in order to better manage the rigors of high-intensity training and maintain optimal function.

Many athletes and, sadly, many coaches at every level of competition think higher intensity and more volume are the only keys to improving performance. Although both are incredibly important parts of a winning recipe, my experience suggests that interruptions due to avoidable injury have a more significant effect on longevity and performance than any particular training protocols. Similar to a targeted approach to static stretching, OSC requires you to carefully identify the areas in your body that are most vulnerable to injury, consider your current level of acute irritation and use that information as a starting point for targeted self-care. Surveying the scene is equally necessary for athletes and sports enthusiasts who perceive themselves as injury-free. Careful self-assessment will increase the likelihood of continued good health and decrease injury interruptions. The techniques listed below represent tools for athletes and exercise enthusiasts to maintain their highest possible levels of physical functioning.

Even a small, consistent commitment to OSC significantly decreases the likelihood of injury and the length of time it takes to recover from relatively minor overuse injuries. The techniques can be done in the comfort of your own home or the designated stretching areas within many fitness facilities. In good weather, I urge the athletes I coach to do their OSC right on the court or playing field after practice, if space allows. YMCAs, Jewish Community Centers (JCCs) and many private fitness facilities are increasingly providing well-equipped and comfortable areas to execute OSC techniques. The Mission Valley YMCA, the Sporting Club in UTC and the La Jolla JCC are facilities that I utilize in my own personal fitness training, and all do an excellent job of providing comfortable space and modern OSC equipment. The Mission Valley YMCA, like a growing number of fitness clubs across the country, has begun blending safe therapeutic tools with traditional fitness equipment, allowing the possibility for optimum health to rise.

OSC typically involves the use of physioballs, tennis balls, soft balls, Styrofoam rollers, hanging bars and therapeutic hot and cold modalities. Such modalities include ice packs, ice massage, ice baths, hot packs, hot baths, and steam rooms or saunas. The use of any hot and cold modalities should first be discussed with your physician.

All of the above tools can be used to either stretch or massage muscles, softening and encouraging them to return to a more comfortable, relaxed and functional state. If used properly, these tools help the athlete recover more quickly and reduce the intensity and duration of inflammation cycles brought on by training. Much the way a warm-up is designed to deliberately and progressively stimulate the body, this element of a cool-down is designed to systematically lower physiological and psychological stimulation to pre-workout levels. This lowering of intensity and increased state of relaxation is often omitted, and as a result, the athlete loses a very potent restorative and natural healing opportunity.

The recent explosion in participation in yoga, tai chi and Pilates demonstrates our frenzied culture's growing appetite for more activities that have a relaxation and centering component. Even a small amount of attention to OSC techniques can have a profound benefit on the mind, body and spirit.

Primary OSC Tools and Techniques

Styrofoam roller:

Supine chest opener

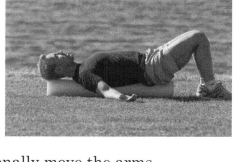

- Rest entire spine and head into the roller.
- Dip chin slightly, avoiding an arch in the neck.
- Allow shoulders and arms to hang gently off the roller.
- In general, keep palms facing up. Occasionally move the arms into a different position along an arc to change the distribution of the stretch across the chest and front shoulder.

Lateral neck stretch

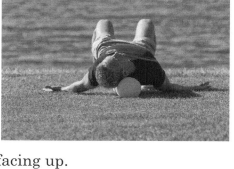

- Rest entire spine into roller.
- Keep knees bent and feet flat on the ground for stability.
- Gently lift head up and off to the left side of the roller.
- Keep one hand behind the neck if your neck needs some support. Otherwise, keep your arms by your side, with palms facing up.
- Eyes gaze out to the left. Jaw and mouth remain relaxed.

Quadriceps

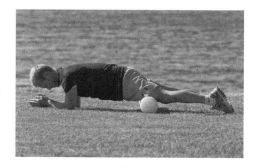

- Lie face-down with the roller across one or both legs, just above the knee.

- Torso should be long, core lightly engaged, shoulder blades drawn slightly in and down, low back mostly flat.
- Slowly move your thighs from side to side over the roller to provide "cross fiber" friction on the front of the thighs.
- After several side-to-side moves, move the roller up a few inches, working the next section of the quadriceps.
- Continue with this pattern until you reach the tops of your quads.
- Depending on your allotted time and the relative tightness in your quads, you can repeat as you make your way back down the leg, stopping just above the knee. Another option is a very slow but more continuous rolling motion from just above the knees to the top part of the quads, with less side-to-side movement.

IT band

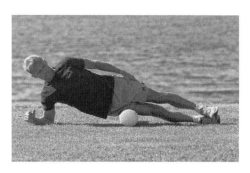

- Start on your right side, with your right elbow lined up underneath your right shoulder.
- Your entire torso and neck should be long and in alignment.
- Place roller just above the knee on the outside of the right leg.
- Keep your core lightly engaged throughout and allow your weight to drop down into the roller as you very slowly move your body over the roller.
- You can lean in or slightly out to focus your body weight into different aspects of the IT Band.
- Note: This will be uncomfortable but not unbearable. Use your upper body and body position to put only as much pressure as your leg can tolerate and assimilate. At most, it should cause a "hurts so good" sensation.

Thoracic back bends

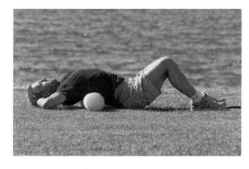

- Lie face-up with the roller across the upper thoracic area of your spine, just below the shoulder blades.
- Place your hands behind your head for gentle support of the neck if you head does not lie comfortably on the ground.
- Extend your legs or bend your knees to get more or less pressure into the upper back.
- Allow your upper back to bend and your chest to open as you continue to breathe comfortably.
- Note: For some people, the standard foam roller may be too big a tool to start with. A tightly folded beach towel or tightly rolled yoga mat in the same position will provide a milder back bend and can be used as a transition to the roller back bend.
- Slow movement down towards the middle and lower end of the back can be added if you are using the roller.
- Attempt to transfer the weight of your body broadly into the soft tissue across the back, not into the little bones of the spine.

Tennis ball self-massage:

- Lie on your back in a relaxed position and breathe comfortably.
- Put a firm tennis ball in the area between one of your shoulder blades and your spine.
- Gently roll the ball on any tight spots, allowing your body to sink down into the ball.
- If you feel sharp pain, stop and get off the ball. Reposition yourself.
- Some other common tight spots that respond well to this type of self-massage (myofascial release) are the muscles that run parallel to your spine, the muscles of the outer hip, the calves

(lower legs) and the center of the shoulder blades, though this last area requires that you go even more slowly and exercise more caution, as there is very little soft tissue there.

- A rubber-coated softball or baseball can be used for the thicker muscles of the outer hips and calves if more pressure is needed.
- Remember to apply pressure smoothly and gently into the muscle, not the bone. Often, just lying on the ball without any movement provides good "trigger point" pressure into one spot and can be a method of release.

Physioball:

Supported face-down forward bend

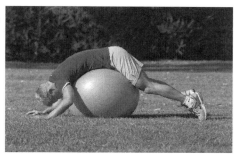

- Allow your body to comfortably melt over the ball.
- Keeping hands and feet in contact with the ground will largely take out the balancing challenge and allow the body to relax into the forward bend.

Supported face up back bend

- Sit on the ball and then systematically roll the ball underneath your back until you feel a comfortable stretch across your chest and the front of your shoulders.
- Arms can be out to the side or above the head. I recommend keeping the palms facing up.
- You can interlock your hands behind your head and provide gentle support to your neck, but do not tug or pull on your neck. It should remain neutral.

Hot and Cold Modalities:
- Heat as part of a pre-practice circulation-enhancing routine
- Cold as part of a post-practice anti-inflammatory routine

I cannot stress enough the importance for individuals and fitness facilities to commit to setting aside adequate space to carry out OSC techniques. In my own home, modest in size by any standard, I keep a couple of OSC tools tucked in a corner in my living room as well as in my home office. On any given evening, while I make my personal phone calls, I execute some of these OSC techniques while talking on a hands-free device to friends and family.

Post-Workout Hydration and Nutrition

An essential and yet commonly overlooked aspect of initiating recovery from a practice or a competition is post-workout hydration and nutrition. Although as athletes we usually experience fatigue, soreness and exhaustion at a broad level of awareness, both exercise and recovery actually begin at the cellular level. Since our cells are between sixty to ninety percent water by weight, hydrating the body after a workout is the first order of affairs, and every individual has different hydration needs and requirements—there is no single prescription for all athletes and fitness enthusiasts. However, water and a combination of carbohydrates and proteins at a roughly 4:1 ratio are essential for optimal recovery in the first thirty minutes after a workout. Such a combination of the macro-nutrition described above supplies the body with the fluids and raw materials needed to repair, rebuild and re-energize the body. I consider nutrition in a larger sense to be the "Sixth Pillar" and I will deal with it comprehensively in an upcoming blog series and book. In the meantime, know that consuming some quality calories immediately after a workout speeds up recovery. Like many of the techniques described in this book, high-quality post-practice nutrition requires planning ahead. If the facility you train at does not have quality nutrition available for purchase, make homemade snacks and have them available in a lunch box or portable cooler in your car.

Epilogue

Nothing in the world can take the place of Persistence. Talent will not; nothing is more common than unsuccessful men with talent. Genius will not; unrewarded genius is almost a proverb. Education will not; the world is full of educated derelicts. Persistence and determination alone are omnipotent. The slogan 'Press On' has solved and always will solve the problems of the human race.

—Calvin Coolidge, 30th president of the United States

Two years after becoming injured in the United States Lifesaving Association National Championships, I arrived in Seal Beach, California, to compete in the Southern California Regional Lifesaving Championships. It was a perfect summer day with a light breeze blowing out of the west. The best lifeguard competitors from all over California, along with competitors from Australia, were present to swim, paddle, run and row for the title of State Champion. This annual regional meet occurred two weeks before the national championships in late July.

Like the summer of '09, my off-season preparation for the 2011 summer competitions had been exemplary. Beginning in January, with a plan to gradually increase intensity and frequency of competition, I had set my pre-summer proximal focus on the 2011 United States Masters Swimming National Championships in Tempe, Arizona, held in early May. Although swimming is my weakest discipline in lifeguard competitions, it is a significant component of my training regimen, because it supports the other aquatic disciplines I love so much, like paddling and kayaking. It also has a very low wear-and-tear factor on the body. By competing in off-season swim meets, I train the same energy delivery systems I rely on when I compete in my preferred discipline, and I keep my competitive juices flowing all year. Although I often finished in the back of the pack in many of my events at the National Masters Swim Meet, it remained an excellent preparation for my summer events. Nothing increases ones fitness level like racing.

As summer came around, I narrowed my focus and raced in four lifeguard competitions. All of these competitions were strategically chosen to prepare me for the State Championships and the National Lifesaving Championship that would be held in Cape May, New Jersey, in August. Although racing too frequently can lead to injury, not racing enough and then expecting the body to perform at the larger meets can also be dangerous.

My once-injured back held up through all these early season competitions with only minimal signs of irritation. The rigorous attention to flexibility, stability and sufficient recovery had fortified my physical foundation. The shift I made to keener body awareness, more sensibility in setting total training volume, and, most importantly, my willingness to do the right thing even when I didn't feel like it, had paid off.

But there I was again, this time at the State Championships in Seal Beach, wrestling with the same issue that I had faced in 2009. I had to decide if I should race exclusively in my age group or tackle the open competition as well. A recreational fitness enthusiast would probably just play it safe, but that, of course, is not me. The thrill of stretching the limits is in my blood. So I decided to take a middle ground and strategically do some of both.

Early in the day, I finished second in the open paddleboard qualifying race, right behind the defending National Champion, Brian Murphy. Fifteen minutes later, I had a second race, an age group final in the paddleboard, where I finished first, earning an age group California State Championship against a highly competitive group, all but one of whom had sat out the open qualifying round. My enthusiasm and fitness level felt fantastic, but the intrinsic muscles of my core were dangerously fatigued. Immediately after I finished the age group championship race, the rational part of me debated whether I needed to race in the open paddleboard final. As I walked towards the starting line, I looked at the younger men, who had been resting for the past thirty minutes. Standing behind the starting line, minutes away from the start of the race, I began a quick review of the goals I had set for the day and measured the potential costs and benefits of racing again in such short order.

I wanted to qualify in the open division, which I did, finishing second behind the U.S. Champion. I wanted to win my age group event, and I did that too. As I looked at the eager and enthusiastic young bucks assembling near the starting line, I realized that if I were fresh, like my younger competitors, a top finish in this race was a definite possibility. But I wasn't. With my fatigue high, I predicted my best finish to be in the middle of the pack.

As I waited for the race to begin, I noticed a dull pain in my lower back and an unusual tightening in my groin. The race officials called us to the starting line. I got up, but paused. Without thinking, I took a couple of steps backwards and sat back down in the sand. I heard the gun go off and watched the race unfold. I had made my choice with a more sensitive and profound awareness of my body than I would have done at any other time in the past. There was a day of racing ahead, and my prudent decision both increased the likelihood of success throughout the day and decreased the likelihood of an injury cycle.

That afternoon, I competed in both the age group and open division Ironman. I won a second California Championship in the age group race and was highly competitive in the open race as well. By day's end, I had participated in ten races, probably as many as any other competitor. Like all competitions, the day ended with multiple long walks from base camp to my car, carrying racing equipment, coolers, and Easy-Up tents. This seemed harder than the races themselves! By the time I finally sat in the driver's seat, air conditioning blasting, ready to make the ninety-minute journey back home to San Diego, I was exhausted. But I was also extremely satisfied with my efforts and the results. Although there was a slight twinge in my lower back, I had stopped short of too much. I certainly was on the edge and had hardly been conservative in my race selection that day, but I had made several decisions that had kept me on the good side of injury.

As I drove home from Orange County, I stopped at a YMCA in Encinitas, CA, about two-thirds of the way home, and hung out in the Jacuzzi, sipping my favorite fluid replacement drink. After my dip in the Jacuzzi got some of the stiffness out, I headed to the Y's self-care room for a few minutes of stretching before finishing the ride home and getting to a post-race celebration. I certainly stretched and tested my limits that day, but my preparation supported my choices. The mindfulness I exhibited in picking my races carried the day, and I knew that such mindfulness would have to increase in the years ahead if I was to go the distance.

The lessons I learned while negotiating my back pain, rehabilitating, and reordering how I assess my own limitations forever changed my life. I was reminded once again that life, our bodies, and the activities and people that we love are precious and not to be taken for granted. Having experienced loss at a very young age—the sudden death of my father from a heart attack—I was no stranger to this truth. As I looked back at my previous approach to my training, I recognized that there had been significant cracks in my mental armor and in my physical preparation, important areas that had not been sufficiently developed for a variety of reasons. Oftentimes, many of us look at our circumstances, especially those that are painful, and think how unlucky we are. But to use a cliché, we really are responsible for creating our own luck.

In fact, when it comes to our physical bodies, our athleticism and our relative health, luck is actually a small player in comparison to the many little and not-so-little choices we make. Doing the right things and choosing healthy habits don't guarantee anything, but together they hugely increase the likelihood of long-term success. Such a disciplined commitment, at least, leaves you with the satisfaction of knowing you did your best to control the controllable and take responsibility for your circumstances.

If you have been plagued by overuse injuries and find yourself in an injury cycle, the foundation laid out in this book is one solid first step to taking back control of your health. If executed consistently, the strategies I recommend will fortify your physical foundation and improve your ability to respond constructively when faced with orthopedic challenges.

My hope is that the information in *Going the Distance* provides you with a compass to navigate the journey of the lifelong athlete. Most importantly, it's my hope that my story and the mistakes I have made and victories I have achieved give you an appetite for the transformational power of my personal motto, "Small consistent change, over a significant period of time, leads to Monumental Results."

Train smart, have fun, and never give up!

Coach Cris

For more tips and candid interviews and blog posts, visit the following sites:

goingthedistancebook.com
monumentalresults.com
facebook.com/monumentalresults
youtube.com/monumentalresults

You can also find me on Twitter as @CrisD_Fitness and on Google+ as +Cris Dobrosielski.

Special Thanks

I would like to first thank Larry Rothstein for collaborating with me on all aspects of this book. The countless hours we spent generating and sifting through the stories and the science included in this book were essential. Larry's wisdom and sensitivity encouraged me to stay the course. We will be friends for life and united as lifelong Boston Celtics fans.

Secondly, I would like to thank Alan Traylor, my editor, who came on board in the fourth quarter of this project. His steadiness, insight and complete commitment to the spirit of this book helped me finish strong.

Thanks to Paul Stricker, MD, Stewart Sanders, DPT, Jay Gerzmehle, CHT, and Eric Nielsen, triathlon coach, for their help as technical editors. Their willingness to share their expertise was a key component in the scientific foundation of this book. Thanks also to Peter McCall, M.S., exercise physiologist, from the American Council on Exercise, for his assistance with technical research for this book.

Thanks to Mike Lewis of Ola Vista Photography for capturing the great "ITA", in the moment, shots on both covers and for his detailed work on all of the interior images. Also to Marc "Pops" Balanky for the eleventh hour head shot image on the back cover, you are a fine professional and a loyal friend.

My deepest gratitude goes to my lifelong friend and emotional *consigliore* throughout this entire project, DJ Cannava, for his tireless support and willingness to be available for me No Matter What.

Lastly, to the thousands of individuals, teams and organizations who have trusted and welcomed me into their lives to provide guidance as a trainer and coach. I deeply appreciate the privilege of accompanying you on your journeys and learning with you as you improve your health and your lives.

Made in the USA
San Bernardino, CA
31 August 2014